MENTAL AND SOCIAL DISORDER IN SUB-SAHARAN AFRICA

Recent Titles in
Contributions in Afro-American and African Studies

MENTAL AND SOCIAL DISORDER IN SUB-SAHARAN AFRICA

The Case of Sierra Leone, 1787–1990

Leland V. Bell

Contributions in Afro-American and
African Studies, Number 147

GREENWOOD PRESS
New York • Westport, Connecticut • London

Library of Congress Cataloging-in-Publication Data

Bell, Leland V.
   Mental and social disorder in Sub-Saharan Africa : the case of
Sierra Leone, 1787-1990 / Leland V. Bell.
     p.   cm.—(Contributions in Afro-American and African
studies, ISSN 0069-9624 ; no. 147)
   Includes bibliographical references (p.) and index.
   ISBN 0-313-27942-X (alk. paper)
   1. Mental illness—Sierra Leone—History. 2. Social psychiatry—
Sierra Leone—History. 3. Sierra Leone—Social conditions.
4. Mental health services—Sierra Leone—History. 5. Kissy Mental
Hospital—History.   I. Title.   II. Series.
RC339.S5B45 1991
362.2'09664—dc20   91-14922

British Library Cataloguing in Publication Data is available.

Library of Congress Catalog Card Number: 91-14922
ISBN: 0-313-27942-X
ISSN: 0069-9624

First published in 1991

Greenwood Press, 88 Post Road West, Westport, CT 06881
An imprint of Greenwood Publishing Group, Inc.

Printed in the United States of America

The paper used in this book complies with the
Permanent Paper Standard issued by the National
Information Standards Organization (Z39.48-1984).

10 9 8 7 6 5 4 3 2 1

For Rachel

Contents

Preface

This book is about mental and social disorder in the West African country of Sierra Leone between the eighteenth century and the present. Over the years, Sierra Leone evolved from a British colony to a nation, becoming an independent country in 1961. Much of this study compares and contrasts trends and developments in mental health care in the colonial era with the patterns of treatment in the period since independence. A unique set of records make it possible to examine the epidemiology of psychiatric illness, the varying psychiatric designations, and the changing characteristics of mental patients in Sierra Leone. The historical evidence, put in a social context, shows that social problems rather than mental illness per se account for the increasingly large number of institutionalized mental patients.

Early in the colonial period, a mental institution, Kissy Lunatic Asylum, was established as a depository for the mentally disordered. Located near Freetown, the prime city of Sierra Leone, the asylum served largely this area but, throughout the nineteenth century, it also received patients from other British West African territories. Most of the hospital's clients suffered from a psychiatric illness, and a significant percentage of them had created some public, largely violent, disturbance. In the decades after World War II, the socially disordered became the predominant element in the institution's clientele.

This transformation reflected a basic demographic change in the wider society: cities developed throughout Sierra Leone, and Freetown swelled in size and population. The societal pressures and pathology common to Africa's urban centers affected Kissy hospital. The institution became a place for persons afflicted with the social maladies of late-twentieth-century urban culture, notably drug addiction, alcoholism, crime, divorce, unemployment, social alienation, and homelessness. Such troubles were exacerbated by the country's general economic malaise; from the 1970s, Sierra Leone experienced severe economic depression.

Other sub-Saharan nations underwent similar developments in mental health care. Colonial authorities needed a place to house persons disturbing the public. A mental institution, a facility providing custody for and control over the mentally and socially distraught, became the basic element of African psychiatry. The asylum experienced limited growth, in part because of the economic austerity but also as a result of the prevailing assumptions about madness in Africa.

Colonial medical observers commonly believed that African societies had an exceptionally low incidence of mental disorder. Sub-Saharan Africa, in their view, was an unsophisticated and primitive area, a place devoid of stress and strife where innocent, largely immature people without ambition lived a carefree existence, oblivious to the attractions and demands of the outside world.

In the twentieth century, this perspective faded, and by the 1960s, the decade of independence for many African nations, a new scientific outlook prevailed. Refuting the old myths about insanity in Africa, African psychiatrists have demonstrated that the mental disorders common to Western nations were also most evident in Africa. Indeed, some recent medical reports have suggested that mental disease is more prevalent in the sub-Saharan region than in the developed world.

Institutional psychiatry represented a foreign element in Africa, an additional factor checking its appeal and development. Within the colonial setting, its therapeutic and curative function remained a minimal concern. Most Africans turned away from its offerings, preferring traditional ways of coping with psychiatric illness. They did not believe that insanity was a disease or a natural disorder; instead they viewed it as a punishment or an attack by an unseen, largely inscrutable and malevolent force, an evil or threatening spirit that had to be neutralized and appeased. A traditional healer, rather than a biomedical doctor, it was felt, knew how to cope with such a problem. A large assortment of traditional healers existed, and they presented vigorous competition to psychiatry. In the colonial era, much suspicion and hostility developed between traditional healers and physicians. In recent times, in Sierra Leone and throughout Africa, the advocates on both sides have come to coexist and cooperate; mutual recognition and respect for the appeals and strengths of both systems prevails.

Only a few historical analyses of psychiatric disorders and care in sub-Saharan Africa exist. Most of the published research on African mental health has utilized a sociological, an anthropological, or a strictly medical or psychiatric perspective. While this study draws on these sources, it remains largely an empirical and descriptive historical presentation based on primary materials, notably the case studies of patients at Kissy Mental Hospital and the papers and records of the hospital and related matters located in the Sierra Leone Public Archives.

The opportunity to engage in research in Africa came when I was awarded a Fulbright to teach at Fourah Bay College, University of Sierra Leone. I am most grateful to the members of the history department at Fourah Bay College, namely Professors Akintola J. G. Wyse, C. Magbaily Fyle, and Gustav H. K. Deveneaux. They generated a warm and genial ambiance that facilitated my work.

I am extremely grateful to Dr. E. A. Nahim, director of Kissy Mental Hospital, and Sierra Leone's only psychiatrist. The research for this book could not have been accomplished without his cooperation, support, and friendship. He provided transportation, gave interviews, arranged visitations with traditional healers, and opened his hospital's records and files to me.

I appreciate also the cooperation of E. M. Turner, director, Sierra Leone Public Archives, and the helpful assistance of Kai Lawrence Bockarie, repository clerk, and Sufianu R. Cole, archives stenographer. Professor John C. Burnham, history department, Ohio State University, read the entire manuscript; the incorporation of his criticism into this study has elevated its quality. The staff of the Hallie Q. Brown Library at Central State University, Wilberforce, Ohio, particularly Janet English, interlibrary loan officer, proved a most helpful resource, providing me with materials from faraway libraries and institutions.

MENTAL AND SOCIAL DISORDER IN SUB-SAHARAN AFRICA

1 Introduction

Until recent times, Western observers held that mental illness was an exceedingly rare disorder among Africans. This view stemmed from a prevailing romantic, Rousseauist notion that the cultures of the sub-Sahara were primitive, innocent societies free from the cares and stresses of the industrial order of the West. Here, in Africa, the myth held, people lived in a state of nature and rarely experienced any debilitating mental disorders. Insanity came only with civilization. A sophisticated advanced Western society, it was argued, offered opportunities to individuals and brought them a beneficent standard of living. But civilization also generated tense and compelling pressures and drives for power and success, which caused frequent outbreaks of madness.

Throughout the nineteenth century, travellers and explorers spun variations on these themes: Westerners faced increasing overloads of stressful problems and situations; Africans remained happy members of carefree, simple communities. The varying styles of life and culture presumably accounted for the high incidence of mental illness found in the West and the infrequent occurrence of madness in Africa.

Around 1880, such views were reinforced by another assumption, a social Darwinian notion that the African was an underdeveloped being, a person without intellectual sophistication who had not evolved sufficiently, either culturally or physically, to experience the pain of emotional distress. The African was a relic of the paleolithic age, a childlike savage, impulsive and superstitious, without a culture, a migrant who wandered and fought others; in short, a being arrested in the early evolutionary development of humanity. In any event, most Europeans believed that the African, as either a representative of retarded human evolution or a product of an uncivilized culture, knew little about and rarely experienced mental disturbance.

MEDICAL OBSERVERS IN THE COLONIAL PERIOD

These popular assumptions were echoed in the reports of medical observers for generations. In 1895, T. Duncan Greenlees, medical superintendent of Grahamstown Asylum, South Africa, maintained that investigating the "mental characteristics of savage and semi-savage races" was a most difficult undertaking. He commented, however, that Africans had a "simple mode of life"; they had "no cares and no struggle for existence such as found in European cities." They lived "in the open air, in a perfect climate, with plenty of simple and natural food"; and in this environment, "diseases originating in mental worry and anxiety" were almost nonexistent. Greenlees also argued that the brain of the African was analogous to the "European child's cerebrum," and that the "mental attributes" of the African were "similar to those of a child." And he had apparent epidemiological evidence relating inadequate mental capacity to a behavior disorder. A high percentage of the inmates at his asylum suffered from mania, a condition he ascribed to inferior mental capacities: mania, he claimed, was prevalent "among natives of low developed brain-function."[1]

Around 1910, in another report, a British physician, R. Howard, describing some of the cases of mental illness he encountered over an eleven-year period practicing in southeast Africa, the area near Lake Nyasa, noted that the patients were full of fears and superstitions and, like all stereotypical Africans, had "an undisciplined emotional temperament."[2] Similar findings came out of a study of mental disturbances among West African troops before and during World War II: Africans were depicted as "highly superstitious" and "easily excited" persons who enjoyed simple pleasures and had few needs. Hysteria was the most common psychiatric disorder. According to this report, the intelligence of the soldiers was at the level of a 10-year-old, and emotionally they "may be safely compared with schoolboys." Endowed with such an intellectual and emotional makeup, African troops had to be handled tactfully, in a manner appropriate to restraining unruly adolescents. Simple, clear instructions, along with some flattering remarks, maintained discipline and control.[3]

Expert medical observers shared this general perspective. During the 1930s, for example, particularly influential publications came from a group of colonial physicians, notably H. L. Gordon, J. H. Sequeira, and F. W. Vint, who were identified as the "East Africa School." While serving as officers in East African colonial administrations, chiefly in Kenya, these men conducted anatomical studies, measuring and comparing African and European brains. They declared that the African had a smaller, simpler brain than the European, which accounted for the responsible behavior of the European and the immaturity of the African.[4]

Over time, this racial determinism was blunted: the findings of the East Africa School were shown to be incorrect, misleading, and untenable. Yet some Western physicians, without reference to any deficiencies or inadequacies of the African personality, simply made terse comments that mental disorder was a most uncommon facet of African life. At Lambarene, for example, Albert Schweitzer noted that psychiatric illness was far less frequent in the Congo than in Europe.[5] These remarks were, of course, impressions rather than commentaries based on significant fieldwork or research.

In the medical literature, a variation of the theme linking insanity to civilization persisted. Numerous reports compared the mental health of westernized Africans with the mental condition of indigenous persons who were far removed from outside contacts. Invariably, observers argued that Africans close to European values and peoples experienced a higher incidence of mental illness than those who remained isolated and aloof from non-African influences.

In a 1936 study of mental disorder in Nyasaland, two British medical doctors, Horace M. Shelley and W. H. Watson, found that schizophrenia occurred with greater frequency among Europeanized Africans than among native peoples. Moreover, the largest bloc of inmates at the Zomba asylum, that country's only depository for the mentally ill at the time, came from those tribes having long-standing contacts with European culture.

This report also made a cross-cultural comparison of the types of crimes committed by the criminally insane in Nyasaland, Kenya, and England, concluding that murder was the most common crime among Africans, while larceny prevailed with the English. The authors commented: "this supports the opinion that the nearer one descends to the state of primitive man, the more keen is the desire to kill." Here no distinctions were made among patients of varying degrees of westernization: the presumption was held that the violence of traditional African society, which was typified by tribal wars and hunts for wild beasts, could not be glossed over with a veneer of civilization. The African had been in contact with "civilizing influences" for only a short time, a factor limiting control over his violent "powerful instincts."[6]

In the 1940s, A. C. Howard, a physician in the Colonial Medical Service, recorded his impressions of nervous and mental diseases in Nigeria "gained at the bedside" over a twelve-year period in several African hospitals. He offered some comparisons: the organic psychoses were more evident in Africa than in England, which he attributed to widespread malnutrition as well as the prevalence of such disabling diseases as malaria, pneumonia, and trypanosomiasis. Senile conditions were rare, chiefly because few Africans lived beyond 60 years of age; mania remained a common affliction, and depressive disorders were infrequent.

But Howard provided the beginnings of a more dynamic interpretation. He contrasted the behavioral patterns of patients of differing backgrounds, observing that "the most primitive, uneducated" African experienced hysteria and obsessional states; on the other hand, he noted, "the more highly educated" African succumbed to bouts of anxiety. This condition, he believed, was the result of the intense inner conflict experienced by the westernized African, a person caught between two cultures who struggled to maintain a balance between the rationalism of the West and the values of traditional Africa.[7]

Such cultural conflict received much attention from J. C. Carothers, a medical officer in charge of Mathare Mental Hospital, Kenya. Recognized as an expert on the psychology of Africans, he later interviewed Mau Mau detainees and became an observer for the World Health Organization. In his controversial writings, he expressed some of the sentiments of the earlier physicians of the East Africa School. Carothers depreciated and stereotyped Africans, seeing them as superstitious people bound to ancient beliefs and traditions who remained at a tribal stage of development and held to an illogical or prelogical thought style. They were, in his view, limited, like children, to "phantastic" thinking and daydreaming, to an "immature mode of thought." Their manner of perception, Carothers continued, encouraged an anthropomorphic view of life that blurred distinctions between wish and reality and between thought and imagination.

Carothers did admit that Africans lived in a most difficult physical environment, a setting ridden with disease and widespread malnutrition. On the other hand, he described their social milieu as utopian. Echoing the impressions of nineteenth century travellers, he insisted that Africans thrived in the warm, communal atmosphere of the village, a place free of stress and competition. In these apparently ideal surroundings, insanity occurred rarely, due to "the absence of problems in the social, sexual, and economic spheres" of life. Such difficulties, however, were rampant in Europe and America, and contributed to a high incidence of madness there.

The mental disturbance of the Africans began, Carothers believed, when they moved beyond their tribal boundary and lost the protective social shield of traditional society. Exposed to the aggressive rivalry of the modern world, the individual had an identity breakdown and experienced the pain of detribalization, a condition that could lead to psychotic disruption. In the words of the report: "so long as an African remains at home he is very unlikely to be certified insane, but as soon as he leaves his home his chances of being so certified are much increased." This study concluded that the highest rates of insanity occurred among the most detribalized persons and ethnic groups.[8]

A few writers dissented from the usual discussions of the incidence of mental illness among Africans. Some challenged the view that psychosis was more evident in detribalized or westernized Africans than in the rest of the population. In a 1938 report on the care and treatment of mental patients in Nigeria, R. Cunyngham Brown, a British physician, observed that the same proportion of mentally ill persons occurred in both rural and urban areas. This finding was based on data acquired from his tour of varied regions of the country; Brown found no concrete evidence to support the "clash of culture" theory, the notion that insanity increased wherever African and European values and institutions met and competed or collided.[9]

Another British colonial physician, Geoffrey Tooth, in a study of mental disorder in the Gold Coast, also questioned the assumption that Western demands and values generated anxiety among Africans. While noting that a great gulf separated the educated African from the illiterate peasant, he argued that special circumstances made it appear that the literate person was prone to madness. The data of this study, he emphasized, came from an urban part of the country inhabited by many educated people. In a densely populated area, a psychotic would be noticeable; and Tooth argued that the psychoses took a more dramatic antisocial form among literate Africans. Such factors made the educated mad person more prominent and unacceptable, and implied that literacy, a measure of westernization, contributed to an individual's mental distress.[10]

Late in the colonial period, during the 1950s, C.G.F. Smartt, a
British psychiatrist at Mirembe Mental Hospital, Tanganyika, introduced a curious twist to the debate over the impact of Western
values on the African. Like Carothers, he assigned largely negative attributes to the subject of his study, "the average rural native of Tanganyika." He described this person as "unintelligent,
emotionally unstable, and essentially lazy," a characterization
Smartt muted with the suggestion that the wide prevalence of
malnutrition and infectious diseases may have influenced the
mental development of the East African. A decade earlier, in
Nigeria, A. C. Howard made a similar observation. But Smartt
added a further imputation: the African had not developed a high
standard of morality.

The African's underdeveloped moral standard was attributed by
Smartt to the restrictive nature of African culture, as well as a
possible physical defect. Here Smartt, like earlier observers, gave
some credence to an alleged structural difference between African
and European brains, implying that an anatomical anomaly in the
African could produce psychopathic tendencies. Yet he stressed
that the African had a capacity for development and admitted that
if no neurophysiological difference existed - if African and European brains were the same - the African could "make good" by
acquiring a Western education.

This point was confirmed by the experience of Africans in the
West Indies, where many received a sophisticated education. An
established pattern of training became a part of that culture,
Smartt maintained, and resulted in fewer distinctions between the
personality development of the African and the European. In the
underdeveloped society of East Africa, however, there were few
educated Africans, which made the differences separating natives
and outsiders appear sharper.

Smartt's study concluded with expressions of openness and
tolerance largely missing from the observations of Western
physicians. Alert to the problems of insufficient information and
cross-cultural misunderstanding, Smartt warned of the dangers of
using the assumptions of Western psychopathology to interpret
African behavior. While the African could appear psychotic to
the European, Smartt curtly remarked, the European may seem
"equally psychopathic through the eyes of the rural African in the
bush."[11]

Certain themes emerge from this sample of writings on the insane and on mental illness in colonial sub-Saharan Africa. From
Greenlees in 1895 to Smartt in 1956, each report confirmed the

prevailing notion that madness was a minor health problem in Africa. Mental illness occurred, but with less frequency than found in Western societies. These studies also showed African mental patients succumbing to particular types of mental disturbance: schizophrenia was the most common psychiatric disorder. Most writers agreed that mania was prevalent, but that depressive disorders were rare. Organic psychoses, delirium, and acute confusional states were reported. There were also cases of epilepsy and mental retardation; only a few persons were diagnosed as sufferers of hysteria, anxiety states, or obsessional neurosis. A large number of patients received no classification.

While these observations were based largely on the records of mental hospital inmates, and purported to be the findings of scientific investigations, most of the studies contained a mix of unproved impressions and presumptions. Above all, an underlying notion permeated the literature: Africa was a primitive place, a natural and restricted world with a backward social order, where people of paleolithic mentality existed at a simple level and vented their instincts. This view was an expression of innocent longing for, or a romantic vision of, a primeval utopia. At the same time, it affirmed a colonial bias, and in a most derogatory and condescending manner, promoted a caricature, a racial stereotype, of Africans and their society.

THE END OF COLONIALISM

During the 1960s, the decade of independence for many African countries, the polemics found in earlier colonial studies faded, and a more global and African perspective on mental health issues emerged. Based on new epidemiological, diagnostic, and etiological research, this view showed that many developments in African psychiatric treatment and care, as well as the types of African mental disorders and rates of African mental illness, ran parallel to those seen in the First and Third Worlds.

Some of the evidence that facilitated the change in outlook came from the work of African psychiatrists. T. Adeoye Lambo, for example, a Nigerian psychiatrist, demonstrated that there was no concrete basis for the major assumptions of Carothers, notably the belief that African "backwardness" had a biological foundation, in that it was linked to "frontal idleness." Carothers had stated that "the resemblance of the leucotomized European to the primitive African is, in many cases, complete." And he had argued also that the "normal African mentality" was basically psychopathic. These were gross generalizations based on incomplete and anecdotal evidence, Lambo asserted, and they represented a common reaction of observers baffled by the problems of interpreting behavior in diverse African societies.

Lambo stressed that culture rather than race determined psychological differences between groups. His findings were based on research conducted in the western region of Nigeria, the area of the Yoruba. Here most of the major psychoses and neuroses were seen. Cultural factors, however, could obscure or militate against certain mental disorders. A widespread acceptance of supernaturalism, unrestricted emotionality, ritual dances, and trances might prevent depression and an accumulation of stress, yet provoke anxiety and acute psychotic states. [12]

Along with undermining colonial assumptions, data in the new medical literature demonstrated that a high frequency of mental disorder prevailed throughout Africa. [13] In the 1960s in western Nigeria, an international team of psychiatrists conducted epidemiological research among subjects from cities and villages, and found a high percentage of psychiatric symptoms. These results were compared with the findings of a corresponding research project completed in Canada, and showed a striking similarity regarding both patterns and prevalence of mental illness. [14]

A 1969 study carried out in Ethiopia disclosed significant psychiatric morbidity in rural and urban areas of the country. The authors personally interviewed a random sample of patients from a teaching hospital in Addis Ababa and another nonselected group from a provincial hospital. They discovered that larger numbers of persons suffered more from psychiatric disorders than from infectious diseases. This was an unexpected finding for Africa, where medical planning and thought have been predominantly concerned with regulating communicable disease. [15] Other surprising results came out of medical fieldwork conducted in two small villages in rural Uganda. Here a high level of psychiatric morbidity was discovered, a prevalence twice that found in southeast London. And a notable finding appeared: many persons were affected with depression. [16]

During the preindependence period, depressive disorders were presumed to be absent from African cultures. Several explanations for this apparent rarity were offered by colonial medical administrators. The prevailing assumption was that guilt feelings, self-deprecatory attitudes, sadness, and withdrawn behavior could not develop in the African, a person lacking maturity and a sense of responsibility. Further, since depression occurred most often in older persons, the short life expectancy of people in African societies made it a rare disorder. Another interpretation was that depressed persons do not receive psychiatric attention because they do not present a threat to family or community, and are tolerated.

The modern belief that depression can take different forms was unknown to earlier practitioners who in consequence did not detect the disorder. In the postcolonial era, however, a flood of studies concluded that affective illness was indeed widespread throughout sub-Saharan Africa. Controversy nevertheless continued about the nature of its symptoms. An articulate and influential group of African psychiatrists has maintained down to the present that depression is common, but that its textbook descriptions of excessive guilt, sadness, and hopelessness do not characterize the typical African depressive; instead, somatic symptoms prevail. Other psychiatrists accept this analysis, but emphasize that new evidence is accumulating that feelings of self-reproach and worthlessness are present in many Africans suffering from affective disorders.[17]

Schizophrenia, the most widely reported psychotic illness in sub-Saharan Africa, also continues to stimulate professional dispute, notably in regard to its prognosis. When mental health workers employ a concept of schizophrenia that includes acute transient reactions, the outcome is excellent. And some medical officers argue that the prognosis for schizophrenia is simply better in developing countries than in the Western world, an opinion still in contention. This view is based on the assumption that a mentally ill person will recover in the tolerant and protective atmosphere of the African extended family.[18]

The transient psychoses remain common in Africa. The name and features of this disorder vary across the continent. In Anglophone Africa it is labeled "acute psychotic reaction," and it may be characterized by such features as hysteria, homicidal behavior, mania, confusion, and paranoid delusion. Its etiology, African psychiatrists now suggest, rests with cultural attitudes, notably the general tolerance of dramatic and emotional reactions to psychological pain and distress. Current medical commentators often connect susceptibility to transient psychoses with a poor health environment, physiological disturbances caused by multiple infections, or with malnutrition, vitamin deficiencies, and the health hazards of living in a poverty-ridden community. And this deprived milieu also contributes, such observers claim, to the many organic psychoses found in Africa.[19]

This brief review of the literature on the prevalence of insanity and the nature of mental illness in modern sub-Saharan Africa reveals certain new trends, quite distinct from the patterns of the colonial period. A most obvious contrast is a higher incidence of mental disorder. Contemporary anthropologists and psychiatrists have destroyed the noble savage stereotype and demonstrated that stress does exist in African societies. The tensions of Western life may not be present, but other kinds of strain, such as varied fears, produce anxiety. Fear of vengeful forces or of envious and angry relatives and neighbors are common experiences that generate emotional pain and pressure. And if a significant level of social tension exists, mental illness caused by stressful living must also prevail.

In addition to affirming a high incidence of mental illness in African societies, recent medical researchers have shown that the major mental disorders recognized by Western psychiatry are found throughout the continent. While important variations may exist, notably in the symptoms, prognosis, and social implications of abnormal behavior, the prevailing evidence indicates that the various types of psychotic illness such as schizophrenia and depression, as well as the psychoneuroses, are as evident in the sub-Saharan regions as in other parts of the world.

Another clear trend, illustrated in the recent writings on African mental health issues, is the appearance of an increasing number of psychopathic cases stemming from drug and alcohol abuse and related problems. This development is part of a global problem, manifested most dramatically in the world's urban centers. It is found almost everywhere, however, and few areas of the Third World can remain untouched by the addiction and abuse spawned by the demand for, and traffic in, drugs.

An increase in suicidal behavior may relate directly to the growing number of chemically dependent persons. While historically the rate of suicide in Africa has been low, more recent research reveals a relatively high suicide rate in Zambia and Uganda. The figure remains small when compared with Europe, but is higher than the number for West Africa.

The same trend is evident regarding drug- and alcohol-related problems: the countries of East Africa report a greater number of incidents than is recorded in West Africa. Throughout the continent, according to late twentieth-century psychiatric literature, the most common drug of abuse is *Cannabis sativa*, or marijuana. It is most popular among school and university students. Several factors clearly contribute to drug and alcohol dependency; many observers claim social causes are the most important. For example, addiction is linked to the breakdown of traditional society. In large urban communities, the individual is removed from traditional values and life-styles and may experience powerful feelings of inadequacy and isolation. Alcohol and drugs may offer relief, an escape from emotionally painful social complications.[20]

CULTURAL CONFLICT ILLNESSES

Related to this development is another theme, foreshadowed by some colonial observations and supported by contemporary investigations carried out in Africa and other parts of the world: an increased incidence of mental illness accompanies rapid sociocultural change.[21] New disorders seem to develop among persons caught between two cultures. Lambo used the term "malignant anxiety" to identity a syndrome related to criminal conduct. It was a mental maladjustment of marginal Africans, those individuals who had repudiated or were rejecting traditional values and had not acquired new ones. This behavior, aggressive and hostile, was exhibited most frequently in places inhabited by transients - labor camps or hastily-constructed shanty towns on the outskirts of cities. In these settings, the order and stability of the traditional village were missing; an amorphous social structure and semiviolent atmosphere prevailed. This kind of insecure milieu was the domain of the marginal African, an alienated person without a cultural identity.

Lambo also took notice of the social and psychological maladjustments of "transplanted African adolescents," those young people who left the traditional village to live in a large metropolitan region. The traditional culture, he argued, eased the transition from adolescence to adulthood by means of varied rituals and ceremonies and by providing hierarchies of class, age, and family. In the city, however, this structured communal and familial order collapsed; without such support, adolescents floundered in a milieu of social disorganization, a setting hazardous to their mental health. Lambo cited evidence from such cities as Dakar, Leopoldville, and Johannesburg that illustrated the mental distress of young people: the data showed a high incidence and prevalence of mental and psychosomatic disorders, as well as growing rates of delinquency, prostitution, gang behavior, and other psychopathic reactions.[22]

Another new cultural conflict illness was identified by Raymond Prince, a medical officer at Aro Hospital in Abeokuta, Nigeria. He used the term "brain fag" to designate a syndrome that occurred largely among young male students at either the secondary school or university level. Brain fag involved intellectual impairment, that is, an inability to concentrate, read, listen, or remember. It was characterized by visual and auditory difficulties; for example, a person might not be able to focus to read a page in a book. There might be somatic complaints, the head and neck might be affected with a burning sensation, and a mood of depression frequently enveloped the individual. Students seemed most susceptible to brain fag during times of intense study, notably before, during, or after a final examination period.

The etiology of this disturbance, Prince surmised, was a fundamental cultural conflict - the imposition of European learning techniques upon the Nigerian personality. The methods of Western education concentrate largely on individual work, responsibility, and organization, with few external sources of support and self-esteem; the basic goal is to develop an independent and self-reliant person. According to Prince, such an emphasis on individualism was alien to Nigerian society, a collectivist order in which the group took precedence over the individual. The family was the most obvious part of the Nigerian social structure, and the interests of any member always remained subordinate to one's obligations to the extended family. Here Prince saw a further source of conflict, in that education became an intensely family affair.

While stress was caused by the fusion of individualistic educational techniques with the group-dependent Nigerian personality, additional psychological tension developed from the emotional burdens placed on an educated member of a family. In other words, a student was a special person to the family, a focus of attention, and his success or failure was linked to the prestige and reputation of the family. Success had tremendous importance and value; failure brought humiliation. In short, a special need to succeed in education was engendered by family pressures, and this drive produced much of the stress that precipitated the symptoms of brain fag.[23]

Some recent research on this disorder largely ignores the cultural conflict thesis of Prince, and concentrates on isolating such specific etiological factors as sleep deprivation and amphetamine abuse. The prevailing consensus is that a vicious cycle of events facilitates the onslaught and maintenance of brain fag: intellectual impairment frustrates the student's efforts at attaining educational goals and ambitions; an anxiety state ensues, which necessitates that the person spend more time studying and less time sleeping; the loss of sleep further impairs cognitive functions, causing a renewal of the cycle.[24]

Another perspective is offered by the unique psychiatric disturbances that mental health workers have found among African expatriates. Some educated persons coming home from the United States or Europe may experience mental distress. A study of Liberian students, for example, showed that after receiving advanced college training or degrees at American universities, they returned to Monrovia and, within a few months, exhibited abnormal behavior. A woman complained of insomnia; she had crying spells and always felt tired; she had symptoms of palpitation, remained weak, and experienced increased perspiration. A young man had bouts of severe abdominal pain, and a physical examination revealed no evidence of organic pathology. He had blackouts and complained about headaches. Another male student, an engineer, had headaches, could not concentrate, and remained irritable.

These three students, the author observed, were experiencing an identity crisis, the pain of cultural conflict, a tense inner struggle between traditional Liberian and modern American values. While studying in the United States, they acquired new goals, habits, and beliefs, most notably a driving work ethic and a need for occupational success. Back in Liberia, they found little opportunity to apply their skills and knowledge, and they became dismayed and disillusioned. Their efforts were not appreciated but were ignored or stymied, or were viewed with indifference, and at times, with hostility. The psychiatric syndrome experienced by the students was called "readaptational anxiety," a condition common among expatriate professionals resuming work in Third World societies undergoing rapid cultural change.[25]

In contrast, a homecoming for some African expatriates became part of the cure for a mental disorder occurring while living abroad. Two women, for example, a Nigerian and a Togoese, had strong European influence in their upbringing in professional families. One was born in London, educated in Nigeria, and returned to England to join her accountant husband. The other woman, a single person, had lived in Paris and London as well as in Togo and in Ghana. When emotionally ill, both women remained strongly influenced by traditional beliefs and seemed immune to Western treatment: ECT (electric convulsive therapy) and the major tranquillizers did not alter their disturbed behavior. Both had received treatment from African healers and were warned about witchcraft spells being placed on them. When they became mentally disturbed in London, this admonition was recalled and the women presumed that bewitchment had caused their mental sickness. Both cases had a satisfactory outcome when the women returned to Africa and received treatment from traditional healers.[26]

In a study on mental health and change in East Africa, separation from family and ethnic group was identified as a major factor creating emotional strain. In Uganda, this situation was most apparent in two very different groups - refugees and college students. Migrants came from such nearby countries as the Sudan, the Congo, and Burundi. There were also many "internal wanderers," native Ugandans moving about the country, away from their ethnic region and birthplace. A high percentage of the clients at Butabika Hospital, a Ugandan mental institution, consisted of unemployed persons living alone, isolated from their tribal groups. Lonely immigrants were found to be most prone to mental and physical sickness in a rural community of Buganda, an area of southeastern Uganda.

Significant mental illness also occurred in a large group of students at Makerere University College, Uganda's prime institution of higher education. Here the prevalence rates of psychoses, neuroses, and personality disorders ranked with those of students at the University of Edinburgh and the University of Belfast. While not poverty cases, many in the Makerere group were first-generation college students from traditional rural communities. Observers related the psychiatric illnesses of these students to their separation from home and ethnic group.[27]

Other contemporary researchers investigating the relationship between mental health and rapid sociocultural change in modern Africa have tried to identify the factors that minimize stress and facilitate mental health. The findings of most investigators have shown high rates of psychoses in populations undergoing fast and dramatic change, and have demonstrated that cultural conflict initiates such disorders as malignant anxiety, brain fag, and readaptational anxiety. But it remains clear that some persons and some groups can absorb stress and can adapt positively to a changing social order.

A study of the Serer, a highly traditional people of Senegal, contrasted them in rural and in urban settings, pointing to the factors, chiefly in Dakar, that modified stress and enhanced the successful adjustment of migrants to city living. In line with prevailing research, this study exposed the fallacy of a rural utopia shielding its members from psychopathology. In the village, stress was generated by such problems as a high birth and infant death rate, the prevalence of diseases including malaria and leprosy, exhausted farmland, drought, and a growing population.

On the other hand, Serer living in Dakar transplanted their culture with ease, created an enclave in the city, and policed their own community. These urban residents frowned on extremes of behavior and reminded an offender that "a Serer does not behave like that." Voluntary associations provided migrants with economic aid as well as companionship. Also, adaption to Dakar may have been facilitated by a Serer practice of sending boys away from the family to receive a traditional education. This experience at an early age may have blunted the impact of living alone in Dakar as a young adult.

Along with the conditions and opportunities provided by the Serer culture, each individual brought certain attributes to the migrant situation. An important individual quality, which affected successful adaption, was having an education, especially the ability to read and write French. A Serer, facile in language, the report emphasized, could become bicultural: a person loyal to traditional values and beliefs, but capable of adapting to change and relating to other ethnic groups; in effect, an individual who moved with comfort across cultures, embracing those elements most useful to him. Poor and unskilled migrants, on the other hand, proved most vulnerable to the stresses of a rapidly changing social order.[28]

MENTAL HEALTH INSTITUTIONS

Over the years, then, theorizing about mental illness in Africa has moved from simplistic notions about innocent, stress-free primitive societies to complex analyses of psychiatric disorders in a context of social and transcultural identities and problems. At the same time, African institutional psychiatric care has evolved slowly, and with only limited objectives.

Hospitals for mad persons came with the Western penetration of Africa in the nineteenth and twentieth centuries. Kissy Lunatic Asylum in the British colony of Sierra Leone was the first institution for the insane in sub-Saharan Africa created by a European colonial power. During the nineteenth century, it received mental patients from British West African territories such as the Gambia, the Gold Coast, and Nigeria as well as from Sierra Leone. Throughout much of its history, the Kissy institution remained a custodial facility - a place for the demented and the dangerous, people who were burdens and created trouble for family and society. Along with mental patients, the institution housed various undifferentiated dependents, including paupers, beggars, criminals, the physically maimed and handicapped, and the mentally retarded. In buildings nearby, lepers, the chronic sick, and those afflicted with smallpox were kept isolated.

Later in the nineteenth century, the institution acquired a clearer medical identity and became an integral part of the colonial hospital system in Sierra Leone. A medical officer regularly saw patients, new administrative patterns and regulations for controlling inmates were inaugurated, more efficient record keeping was maintained, and some occupational and recreational therapy occurred. But always the hospital faced difficult, perennial problems: it remained overcrowded and understaffed; it lacked sufficient funding and effective leadership. Clearly, the Kissy hospital was a low priority but a necessary facility, a place designed largely for the custody and control of its clients.

Over time, the Kissy hospital was influenced by the policies and trends of institutional mental health care in the United Kingdom and the United States. After 1945, for example, the electric convulsive therapy, drug treatments, and community care that reigned throughout Western psychiatric institutions formed a major part of the armamentarium of therapeutics at Kissy. Although it was tied to developments in medicine and mental health care in Europe and America, the Kissy hospital was also shaped by the indigenous African culture.

Few Africans accepted the facility as a place to resolve their mental health problems. In Sierra Leone, traditional healers treated and cared for the mentally ill. Mental illness was an inscrutable, highly taboo subject removed from polite discourse and society, a matter kept within the preserve of the extended family. The mental institution was a place of last resort, a building where an incorrigible or lost person was sent when no other option existed.

A related fact limited the hospital's appeal: the nature of its origins and identity. It was an alien facility established by outsiders and designed to serve the needs of the colonial power, chiefly by housing the community's underclass of undesirable, unwanted, and troublesome persons. In short, Kissy Mental Hospital was burdened with varied stigmas: it was a custodial place, a depository for society's rejects; it was a foreign institution, a politically alien place, a colonial establishment; and it was medically and therapeutically removed from African society. Over the years, however, these stigmas may have been softened by the general laxity of the colonial administration, the emerging cosmopolitanism of the Freetown area, and the identification of the Krio, an articulate and influential ethnic group, with the culture and institutions of the United Kingdom.

In 1887, a lunatic asylum opened in Accra, the main city of the Gold Coast. Here developments followed the pattern of Kissy hospital in Sierra Leone. The Accra asylum became an overcrowded facility for the violent and the unfortunate. People took their psychological problems to traditional healers, and the failures of these practitioners went to the asylum. Some therapy may have been offered to the nonviolent and manageable patients who worked at gardening, cleaning, or crafts. Between the world wars, the institution was managed well by a psychiatrist. Under his administration, general conditions improved: some cures were produced; the inmates received adequate food and were kept clean; the hospital provided services to hundreds of clients annually.[29]

Western psychiatric care came in 1907 to Nigeria, the largest British West African area, with the establishment of Yaba Asylum in Lagos. Later, another mental institution was opened in Calabar, and in 1945, Lantoro Asylum, initially established for criminal cases, was opened in Abeokuta. These facilities were largely custodial places of confinement for the antisocial and abandoned - those who were friendless, sick, poor, or elderly. For most Nigerians, active mental health care rested with traditional healers. In 1954, a unique facility, Aro Hospital, in Abeokuta, blended successfully Western and traditional modes of care and treatment. In recent years, Nigeria, having such advantages as a large population, a significant economic and industrial base, and well-established medical training programs, expanded its biomedical psychiatric care to include facilities at general hospitals and at the Universities of Ibadan, Ife, Lagos, Benin, and Ahmadu Bello. Soon after the Nigerian civil war ended, in 1970, a new mental health unit, Anambra State Psychiatric Hospital, opened at Enugu to cope with the war's psychiatric casualties.[30]

In contrast to Nigeria's active policies and programs, most other sub-Saharan countries have remained largely stagnant in mental health care, sustaining decades-old problems and beliefs. Such matters as a general indifference, a lack of funds, an acceptance of traditional healers and views of madness, coupled with a prevailing assumption that mental illness is a minor health problem compared to prominent physiological afflictions, have continued from colonial times to the present. In Zimbabwe, Ingutsheni Hospital opened in 1908, and it served areas embraced by present-day Zambia and Malawi. Another mental institution, Ngomahuru Hospital, emerged from a former leprosarium holding mental patients. A small nervous disorder hospital existed at Bulawayo, along with a Catholic missionary facility for disturbed and abandoned children. Many of the clients at these institutions were vagrants without families.

A similar situation prevailed in Tanganyika, where distraught individuals without relatives, or those unable to remain at home, went to Mirembe Hospital. In 1960, more than 40 percent of this facility's patients were senile or mentally defective. Apparently, as in older European facilities, families found relief from a painful responsibility by sending their difficult dependents to a mental institution.[31]

FEATURES OF AFRICAN PSYCHIATRY

The use of a security force to bring patients to insane asylums was a characteristic feature of colonial care. Police intervention in psychiatric cases remains a common occurrence throughout Africa, although it may be more prevalent in the eastern areas of the continent. In Zambia, for example, over a one-year period, 65 percent of patients sent to a hospital and 58 percent of inmates brought to a psychiatric facility required a security escort.[32]

Colonial and contemporary African psychiatry has been marked also by an insufficient number of trained mental health personnel, a major factor limiting programs and services. Nigeria, with over 100 million people and an active concern for improving and expanding mental health facilities, may have around fifty psychiatrists. Sierra Leone, a country of 4 million, has one psychiatrist. In Zambia, Chainama Hill Psychiatric Hospital has a capacity of over 400 beds, but only a few psychiatrists. Marracuene Asylum, a small institution for dangerous mental patients, was established in Mozambique in 1930. The lack of personnel, however, forced an open-door policy, with inmates leaving and returning at will. Ethiopia remained without a special depository for the mentally ill until 1940, when Ammanuel Hospital, with 150 beds, opened in Addis Ababa. It took seriously disturbed cases only. For the large country of Sudan, an understaffed community clinic operated in Khartoum in the 1950s and served about 5,000 clients annually.

In recent years, there has been a paucity of psychiatric beds and personnel in most of Francophone Africa. Two small facilities in Cameroon, at Yaounde and at Duala, offered fewer than 150 beds. A psychiatric hospital at Bingaville in the Ivory Coast had a capacity of 250 beds. In Niger, Mali, and Burkina Faso, each nation had a ward in a general hospital, the country's only facility for psychiatric care.

Senegal, on the other hand, has provided more developed services. In the colonial era, some mentally distraught Africans were sent to asylums in France. And while the world wars upset plans for constructing a mental hospital in Dakar, the general hospitals did have isolation pavilions and rooms, with cells for mentally ill patients. In 1956, a neuropsychiatric center was created in Dakar, where Henri Collomb conducted significant research in social psychiatry. Collomb favored a team approach - a mix of specialists from different fields and backgrounds - as he went about the study and resolution of the problems of psychiatric care in Senegal.[33]

Kenya, in East Africa, perhaps more than any country, typifies the evolution, nature, and direction of African psychiatry. During the early years of colonial rule, a prison in Mombasa quartered mentally disturbed inmates. Around 1914, a smallpox isolation center was converted into a psychiatric unit and evolved into Mathare Hospital, Nairobi. Eventually, psychiatric beds were provided in general hospitals.

Over the years, the country changed. Many non-Africans came and stayed; communities of Asians as well as Europeans, predominantly English, emerged, and Kenya became a multiracial society. While general tolerance prevailed, racial tensions developed between the English and the Kikuyu, notably in the early 1950s during the Mau Mau disturbances. The English expatriate physician J. C. Carothers based much of his controversial writings and observations about the African personality mostly on data acquired in Kenya.

After independence, in the early 1960s, the problems of mental health common to most of Africa persisted in Kenya. Medical attention focused on communicable and preventable diseases. For many Kenyans, madness was not a medical matter and was best left to the traditional healer; mental health services were limited by a lack of funds, facilities, and personnel. In 1979, nine psychiatrists practiced in Kenya, a nation of fifteen million. There were some psychiatric nurses, but only two clinical psychologists, and no psychiatric social workers. There were plans, however, for new training programs, health education, and the establishment of new community psychiatric units.[34]

In South Africa, unique historical developments, chiefly the growth of a strong economy coupled with a restrictive social system culminating in apartheid, profoundly affected the delivery of psychiatric care. Initially, as in other parts of Africa and the world, insane people received no special care or treatment; they were placed with other sorts of dependents. In the early 1840s, a facility on Robben Island housed an undifferentiated group of the unwanted: lepers, lunatics, paupers, and the chronic sick. Some mentally ill remained at the institution until 1913.

In the twentieth century, South Africa developed with the First World, and by the 1950s had a modern mental health system, with ten state mental hospitals, two restricted to Africans only. In contrast to the rest of the continent, sufficient funds were available and mental health staffs included psychiatrists, trained nurses, social workers, and clinical psychologists.

Weskoppies Mental Hospital, one of the black institutions, held, in 1952, over nine hundred male Bantu patients. The majority of new admissions were cases involving crime, violence, and vagrancy. A significant number of patients also were affected by syphilis (often a serious cause of mental illness), alcoholism, and malnutrition. Almost all of the newly admitted were young men, and many were discharged, sufficiently recovered, within six months. The readmission rate was low. In recent years, the conditions and standards of the hospital, already poor in the 1950s when compared with other South African mental institutions, deteriorated further with the intensification of apartheid.[35]

Basic differences still distinguish mental institutions in Africa from their counterparts in the West, especially in England and the United States. The early nineteenth century Western insane asylum was, in most instances, a retreat, a hopeful place for the mentally ill, a refuge enveloped with an atmosphere of confidence and optimism. A basic assumption prevailed: when patients received the proper care - a therapeutic regimen known as moral treatment - they would be cured and returned to society. By the 1870s, moral treatment faded, and the asylum became a large, overcrowded institution with custodial and welfare roles.

The therapeutic ideal and rhetoric, however, persisted. At times, political, reformist, and medical pressures militated against the mere warehousing of patients and brought change, transforming the asylum into a hospital and later into a mental health center.

In Africa, mental institutions never really acquired a major therapeutic role. No one in the community exposed abuses or demanded reform and innovation. Moral treatment was not transported to Africa. In the 1840s, while the insane went with varied social dependents and outcasts to Kissy in Sierra Leone and Robben Island in South Africa, moral treatment set the tone for the practice of institutional care in England and in the United States.

The colonial asylum in Africa assumed major police and welfare functions. Above all, reminiscent of Michel Foucault's description of the confinement policies of eighteenth century France,[36] the African mental hospital became an institution for social control - a depository for keeping the deviant, the criminal, the troublesome, the sick, the unwanted, the transient, as well as the insane off the streets. Throughout its history, this role remained paramount.

By the 1930s, most of the European colonies in Africa maintained mental institutions that had adopted the outward features, chiefly the psychiatric terminology and organization, of Western facilities. The hospital clientele, however, revealed the main purpose and nature of African institutions. The majority of patients did not end up there to be cured of mental disorder - they had created some socially disruptive problem that required their incarceration and isolation from the community.

Psychiatry in Africa did not fully benefit from the dramatic advances of Western medicine. Until the late nineteenth century, European medicine, lacking expertise, knowledge, and motivation, intervened in Africa only in a limited way, largely to control such long-standing, familiar, and threatening afflictions as smallpox, leprosy, and lunacy. While vaccination attacked smallpox, segregation contained leprosy and lunacy. In most instances, the sufferers of these disorders were kept within a cluster of small buildings in an isolated area.

By 1900, Western medicine had acquired increased prestige and power. Its practitioners were well-trained professionals, the products of respected medical schools. Physicians exploited new techniques, such as microscopy and chemical analysis, which allowed them to identify disorders with greater sophistication and awareness. New areas of interest, such as sanitation and public health, along with developing specialties, including bacteriology, had obvious applications in the colonial world. Tropical medicine burgeoned; schools of tropical medicine were opened in the United Kingdom, on the Continent, and in the United States.

At the opening of the twentieth century, modern medicine, confident and aggressive, had become imperial: it established and maintained strong links between the European capital and the colonial regions. It sent out specialists, created health commissions, and directed campaigns to eradicate such diseases as sleeping sickness, cholera, yellow fever, and malaria.[37]

Psychiatry was not part of this effort; it may have gained only indirectly or vicariously, in that it was identified as a specialty within Western medicine. Expatriate colonial administrators and medical officers accepted the prevailing notions about the general absence of mental illness in African societies. And most Africans remained confident that traditional healers could best help resolve problems of mental disturbance.

NOTES

1. T. Duncan Greenlees, "Insanity Among the Natives of South Africa," *Journal of Mental Science* 41 (1895): 71-79.

2. R. Howard, "Emotional Psychoses Among Dark-Skinned Races," *Journal of Tropical Medicine and Hygiene* 13 (1910): 169-73.

3. N. Dembovitz, "Psychiatry Among West African Troops," *Journal of the Royal Army Medical Corps* 84 (1945): 70-74. The view of the adult African as a child was also a dominant theme in late-nineteenth century anthropological studies on Africa.

4. H. J. Simons, "Mental Disease in Africans: Racial Determinism," *Journal of Mental Science* 104 (1958): 377-88.

5. Albert Schweitzer, *On the Edge of the Primeval Forest* (London: Black, 1948).

6. Horace M. Shelley and W. H. Watson, "An Investigation Concerning Mental Disorder in the Nyasaland Natives," *Journal of Mental Science* 83 (1936): 701-30.

7. A. C. Howard, "Notes on Nervous and Mental Diseases Encountered in Nigeria," *Transactions of the Royal Society of Tropical Medicine and Hygiene* 41 (1948): 823-28.

8. J. C. Carothers, "A Study of Mental Derangement in Africans, and an Attempt to Explain Its Peculiarities, More Especially in Relation to the African Attitude to Life," *Journal of Mental Science* 93 (1947): 47-86; Carothers, *The African Mind in*

Health and Disease: A Study in Ethnopsychiatry (Geneva: World Health Organization, 1953).

9. R. Cunyngham Brown, *Report III: On the Care and Treatment of Lunatics in the British West African Colonies: Nigeria* (Lagos 1938).

10. Geoffrey Tooth, *Studies in Mental Illness in the Gold Coast* (London: His Majesty's Stationery Office, 1950).

11. C.G.F. Smartt, "Mental Maladjustment in the East African," *Journal of Mental Science* 102 (1956): 441-66. This overview of colonial medical observations touches only some of the available sources in English. For the experience of German practitioners in Africa, see Albert Diefenbacher, *Psychiatrie und Kolonialismus: Zur "Irrenfürsorge" in der Kolonie Deutsch-Ostafrika* (Frankfurt: Campus Verlag, 1985). For French views see Antonine Porot, "L'oeuvre psychiatrique de la France aux colonies depuis un siècle," *Annales Médico-Psychologiques* 101 (1943): 357-78; and Henri Collomb, "Histoire de la psychiatrie en Afrique noire francophone," *African Journal of Psychiatry* 2 (1975): 87-115.

12. T. Adeoye Lambo, "The Role of Cultural Factors in Paranoid Psychoses among the Yoruba Tribe," *Journal of Mental Science* 101 (1955): 239-66.

13. G. Allen German, "Aspects of Clinical Psychiatry in Sub-Saharan Africa," *British Journal of Psychiatry* 121 (1972): 461-79; German, "Mental Health in Africa: I. The Extent of Mental Health Problems in Africa Today. An Update of Epidemiological Knowledge," *British Journal of Psychiatry* 151 (1987): 435-39.

14. T. Adeoye Lambo, "Neuropsychiatric Observations in the Western Regions of Nigeria," *British Medical Journal* 2 (1956): 1388-94; Lambo, "Further Neuropsychiatric Observations in Nigeria," *British Medical Journal* 11 (1960): 1696-1704; A. M. Leighton, T. A. Lambo, C. C. Hughes, D. C. Leighton, and D. B. Macklin, *Psychiatric Disorder Among the Yoruba* (Ithaca, N. Y.: Cornell University Press, 1963).

15. R. Giel and J. N. Van Luijk, "Psychiatric Morbidity in a Small Ethiopian Town," *British Journal of Psychiatry* 115 (1969): 149-62.

16. John Orley and John K. Wing, "Psychiatric Disorders in Two African Villages," *Archives of General Psychiatry* 36 (1979): 513-20.

17. M. J. Field, "Mental Disorder in Rural Ghana," *Journal of Mental Science* 104 (1958): 1043-51; Raymond Prince," The Changing Picture of Depressive Symptoms in Africa," *Canadian Journal of African Studies* 1 (1968): 177-92; Morton Beiser, "A

Study of Depression Among Traditional Africans, Urban North Americans, and Southeast Asian Refugees," in Arthur Kleinman and Byron Good, eds., *Culture and Depression* (Berkeley: University of California Press, 1985), 272-98; German, "Aspects of Clinical Psychiatry," 469-72; G. Allen German, "Mental Health in Africa: II. The Nature of Mental Disorder in Africa Today. Some Clinical Observations," *British Journal of Psychiatry* 151 (1987): 441-42.

18. German, "Aspects of Clinical Psychiatry," 467-69; German, "Mental Health in Africa," 440-41; Adebayo Olabisi Odejide, Lamidi Kolawole Oyewunmi, and Jude Uzoma Ohaeri, "Psychiatry in Africa: An Overview," *American Journal of Psychiatry* 146 (1989): 711-12.

19. German, "Aspects of Clinical Psychiatry," 465-67; German, "Mental Health in Africa," 442-43; Odejide, Oyewunmi, and Ohaeri, "Psychiatry in Africa," 712; Wolfgang C. Jilek and Louise Jilak-Aall, "Transient Psychoses in Africans," *Psychiatrica Clinica* 8 (1970): 337-60.

20. German, "Mental Health in Africa," 442; Odejide, Oyewunmi, and Ohaeri, "Psychiatry in Africa," 712; Charles R. Swift and Tolani Asuni, *Mental Health and Disease in Africa: With Special Reference to Africa South of the Sahara* (Edinburgh: Churchill Livingstone, 1975), 120-27. The comments here are restricted to what appears in the psychiatric literature.

21. George M. Foster and Barbara Gallatin Anderson, *Medical Anthropology* (New York: Wiley, 1978): 93-96.

22. T. Adeoye Lambo, "Malignant Anxiety: A Syndrome Associated with Criminal Conduct in Africans," *Journal of Mental Science* 108 (1962): 256-64; T. A. Lambo, "Adolescents Transplanted from Their Traditional Environment: Problems and Lessons out of Africa," *Clinical Pediatrics* 6 (1967): 438-45.

23. Raymond Prince, "The Brain-Fag Syndrome in Nigerian Students," *Journal of Mental Science* 106 (1960): 559-70.

24. O. Morakinyo, "A Psychophysiological Theory of a Psychiatric Illness (the Brain-Fag Syndrome) Associated with Study Among Africans," *Journal of Nervous and Mental Disease* 168 (1980): 84-89; Olufemi Morankinyo, "The Brain-Fag Syndrome in Nigeria: Cognitive Defects in an Illness Associated with Study," *British Journal of Psychiatry* 146 (1985): 209-10; Brian Harris, "A Case of Brain-Fag in East Africa," *British Journal of Psychiatry* 138 (1981): 162-63. Brain fag is identified often as neurasthenia, a disorder appearing in the late nineteenth-century West, especially in the United States. The diagnosis persisted in European psychiatry long after it left America.

25. Ronald M. Wintrob, "A Study of Disillusionment:

Depressive Reactions of Liberian Students Returning from Advance Training Abroad," *American Journal of Psychiatry* 123 (1967): 1593-97.

26. Anne E. Farmer and Wojciech F. Falkowski, "Maggot in the Salt: the Snake Factor and the Treatment of Atypical Psychosis in West African Women," *British Journal of Psychiatry* 146 (1985): 446-48.

27. M. Assael and G. A. German, "Changing Society and Mental Health in Eastern Africa," *Israel Annals of Psychiatry and Related Disciplines* 8 (1970): 52-74.

28. Morton Beiser and Henri Collomb, "Mastering Change: Epidemiological and Case Studies in Senegal, West Africa," *American Journal of Psychiatry* 138 (1981): 455-59.

29. E.F.B. Forster, "A Short Psychiatric Review from Ghana," in *Mental Disorders and Mental Health in Africa South of the Sahara* (Geneva: World Health Organization, 1958), 37-41; K. David Patterson, *Health in Colonial Ghana: Disease, Medicine, and Socio-Economic Change, 1900-1955* (Waltham, Mass.: Crossroads Press, 1981): 82-83.

30. A. Ordia, "A Brief Outline of the History and Development of Mental Health Services and Facilities in Nigeria for the Care and Treatment of Mentally Ill Patients," in *Mental Disorders and Mental Health*, 50-51; T. Asuni, "Aro Hospital in Perspective," *American Journal of Psychiatry* 124 (1967): 763-70; Ralph Schram, *A History of the Nigerian Health Services* (Ibadan: Ibadan University Press, 1977), 207-10, 382, 386-89; Anja Forssen, "Psychiatry in Nigeria," *Psychiatric Annals* 8 (1978): 311-14; Olayiwola A. Erinosho, "The Evolution of Modern Psychiatric Care in Nigeria," *American Journal of Psychiatry* 136 (1979): 1572-75; R. O. Jegede, "Nigerian Psychiatry in Perspective," *Acta Psychiatrica Scandinavica* 63 (1981): 45-56.

31. W. Murdoch, "The Evolution of Psychiatric Care in Zimbabwe," in Olayiwola A. Erinosho and Norman W. Bell, eds., *Mental Health in Africa* (Ibadan: Ibadan University Press, 1982), 28-32; John Iliffe, *The African Poor: A History* (London: Cambridge University Press, 1987), 212; C.G.F. Smartt, "Psychiatry in Tanganyika," in *Mental Disorders and Mental Health*, 59-61, 62-68.

32. Odejide, Oyewunmi, and Ohaeri, "Psychiatry in Africa," 712-13.

33. Ibid., 713; F. B. Hylander, "Summary Information on Mental Disease in Ethiopia," "Mental Hygiene and Mental Health in Mozambique," and T. el Mahi, "Mental Health Work in the Republic of Sudan," in *Mental Disorders and Mental Health*, 35-36, 45-49, 56; David Lippman, "Psychiatry in Ethiopia," *Cana-*

dian Psychiatric Association Journal 21 (1976): 383-88; R. Collignon, "Social Psychiatry in French-Speaking Africa," in Erinosho and Bell, *Mental Health in Africa*, 8-27.

34. E. L. Margetts, "Psychiatric Facilities in Kenya," in *Mental Disorders and Mental Health*, 42-44; D. M. Ndetei, "Psychiatry in Kenya: Yesterday, Today, and Tomorrow," *Acta Psychiatrica Scandinavica* 62 (1980): 201-11.

35. I. R. Vermooten, "Brief Outline of Facilities in South Africa for the Treatment of the Mentally Ill with Special Reference to the Mentally Ill African," in *Mental Disorders and Mental Health*, 57-8; Iliffe, *The African Poor*, 102-03; Alastair M. Lamont and William J. Blignault, "A Study of Male Bantu Admissions at Weskoppies During 1952," *South African Medical Journal* 27 (1953): 637-39.

36. Michel Foucault, *Madness and Civilization. A History of Insanity in the Age of Reason* (New York: Vintage, 1973).

37. The export of Western medicine to non-European areas of the world has excited much interest. For varied interpretations, see David Arnold, "Introduction: Disease, Medicine and Empire," in David Arnold, ed., *Imperial Medicine and Indigenous Societies* (Manchester: Manchester University Press, 1988), 1-26; Roy MacLeod, "Introduction," in Roy MacLeod and Milton Lewis, eds., *Disease, Medicine, and Empire: Perspectives on Western Medicine and the Experience of European Expansion* (London: Routledge, 1988), 1-18; John Ehrenreich, ed., *The Cultural Crisis of Modern Medicine* (New York: Monthly Review Press, 1978); Thomas Akwasi Aidoo, "Rural Health Under Colonialism and Neocolonialism: A Survey of the Ghanaian Experience," *International Journal of Health Services* 12 (1982): 637-57; Dennis A. Itavyar, "Background to the Development of Health Services in Nigeria," *Social Sciences and Medicine* 24 (1987): 487-99.

2 The Setting

Sierra Leone is a tropical country located along the Atlantic coast in the southwestern part of the West African bulge, bordered to the south by Liberia and to the north and east by Guinea. It is about the size of South Carolina. While there is a steady emigration, the population is growing and stands, in the early 1990s, at around 4 million. Freetown, the capital and largest city, has approximately 320,000 inhabitants.

The Portuguese penetrated the coastal peninsula region, the locale of Freetown, in the mid-fifteenth century, naming the area Serra Loya after the wild lion shape of the mountains. Over the years many varieties of this name occurred - Sierra Lyonne, Sierra Leona, Serrelions, Sierraleon, Serrillioon - but eventually Sierra Leone prevailed.[1] A brisk trade developed between, on the one hand, the coastal peoples, notably the Bullom and Temne, and, on the other side, the Portuguese and varied Europeans. Ivory, gold, beeswax, and, most important, slaves, were exchanged for European metalware, clothes, weapons, and other manufactured goods. By the eighteenth century, with the maturing of the European colonies in the Americas, particularly those based on a plantation economy, the demand for slaves intensified. While the major source of slaves was in the south - in the areas of present-day Angola, Nigeria, and Ghana - around 3,000 slaves were taken each year from the coastal regions of Sierra Leone.

Events in England upset this trade in human flesh. An anti-slavery movement agitated English public life in the last quarter of the eighteenth century. One of its most fervent advocates, Granville Sharp, demonstrated that England was free of the peculiar institution by arranging a test case involving a slave, James Somerset. The court ruled slavery illegal in England, a source of relief for the community of Africans living in London, most of whom were refugees from slavery in the New World. Freedom, however, did not bring jobs; unemployment made life difficult for the "black poor," forcing many to become beggars. During and after the American Revolution, their condition deteriorated when more ex-slaves arrived in England; these persons had accepted a British promise of freedom for deserting their American masters.

The plight of unemployed former slaves caught the attention of Sharp, who, after securing support from Parliament, arranged for the transport to Sierra Leone of over four hundred persons. Leaving England in April 1787, they established a settlement Sharp named the Province of Freedom. This experiment failed. The former London residents came unprepared for the wet season. Rains beat down their shelters; many became sick and died; others deserted; and conflict and violence with local peoples doomed their settlement.

To revive the colony, Sharp, along with his business and anti-slavery associates, William Wilberforce, Thomas Clarkson, and others, created in 1791 the Sierra Leone Company, a private trading organization governed by its directors from London. The settlement was renamed Freetown, and in line with the basic goal of the colony, slavery and the slave trade were prohibited within the territory of the company.

The colony received a major boost when new settlers arrived from Nova Scotia. These were ex-slaves freed by British armies during the American War of Independence and taken to Nova Scotia, where they were promised, but never given land. Thomas Peters, one of their spokespersons, went to England to demand justice from the government; he came in contact with the directors of the Sierra Leone Company, who offered him and his Nova Scotians land in Sierra Leone.

In January 1792, excited about acquiring land in Africa, 1,190 former slaves left Nova Scotia for Sierra Leone. While they did receive land, new troubles and problems disrupted colonial life. The European war between France and England spilled over into West Africa: trade was disrupted, prices rose, and a French naval squadron bombarded Freetown. Its sailors sacked the community, burned down all company buildings, and captured its ships.

This was a devastating loss, a setback from which the company never recovered. The community was rebuilt, but a company tax on land angered many Nova Scotians, who assumed that their land was free. An uprising ensued, which the company put down with the aid of a new group of settlers known as the Maroons. They were former rebellious Jamaican slaves the company had brought to Sierra Leone. Originally, many of them were Ashanti from Ghana.

Another serious conflict developed between settlers and local people over land use and ownership - in effect, a dispute over African and English views of land. According to Temne law and custom, outsiders were never given land forever, and when a landlord died, a new agreement was made. The settlers took the opposite position, basing their argument on English law, which accepted a treaty as an absolute agreement. Whenever a land issue arose, the Sierra Leone Company, for example, referred to the Treaty of 1788, negotiated between settlers and local rulers, as a binding agreement that could not be nullified simply by the death of a signatory. Soon after a new Temne ruler emerged in the 1790s, the company refused to draw up a new arrangement, and hostilities broke out. A state of war prevailed, and a series of violent clashes kept the atmosphere tense for several months. It was not until after 1807 that a new treaty, highly favorable to the settlers, was accepted by the Temne. It gave most of the peninsula to the Sierra Leone Company. This represented a hollow victory; by this time, the company was financially depleted and unable to support the settlement. On January 1, 1808, Freetown and the surrounding area became a British Crown Colony, under the king of Great Britain.

THE EMERGENCE OF KRIO CULTURE

Sierra Leone soon acquired major significance in the British assault on the slave trade. Parliament had passed the Anti-Slave Trade Act in 1807, outlawing the trade in British colonies as well as forbidding British subjects to engage in it. Newly established courts in Freetown tried slavers and disposed of slave ships taken by British naval patrols off West Africa. Freetown therefore became a place of liberation for slaves recaptured by the British.

These individuals became known as "recaptives" or "liberated Africans." Many of them were Yoruba from Nigeria; others came from areas such as the Congo, Senegal, and the interior of Sierra Leone. This heterogeneous ethnic mix set them apart from the other, older settlers who looked down on the new immigrants. Unlike the "black poor," the Nova Scotians, and the Maroons - each of whom was partially westernized by experiences in the New World - the recaptives, taken directly off slave ships, had no common language and remained ignorant of Western customs and values. There were conflicts and tensions, and brawls occurred frequently.

Hundreds of recaptives entered the colony each year. By 1815, over 6,000 had arrived; by 1860, around 60,000 had come. Accommodations were quite limited in Freetown. A few served as soldiers in British regiments; some settled and built villages in nearby areas. A community was often named after the place of origin of the settlers, such as Congotown and Kissy; or it received a name from British history, such as Hastings and Waterloo. The colonial government supported missionary work among the recaptives, aiming to westernize and Christianize them. Many were receptive to these efforts: they adopted Christianity, acquired Western names, and identified with the European work ethic. Over the years, with hard work and good luck, they achieved material success.

By mid-century, a new society, Krio culture, had emerged in the colony. The basic elements of the earlier frontier community were gone, for few original settlers remained. Only a trickle of new recaptives entered Freetown. The inland slave traffic did exist, but the Atlantic trade had virtually ended. The divisiveness and suspicion that existed among the ethnic groups had faded, and young people of all groups intermarried, creating a new generation, a fusion of recaptives and settlers. Finally, a lingua franca, Krio, flourished, nurturing relationships and facilitating community integration. Krio culture merged African and Western elements, and it placed strong emphasis on education. Secondary schools operated in Freetown; Fourah Bay College opened in 1827 and became affiliated with the University of Durham in 1876. Some Krios received their higher education and professional training at British universities. A university education brought an individual status along with advancement into the higher levels of society. Over time, a professional class of Krios evolved, many of whom gained distinction in medicine and law as well as education, religion, and administration. Two Krio physicians were specialists in mental disorders. William Awunor-Renner, who practiced around the turn of the century, and M.C.F. Easmon, who worked as a medical officer between 1913 and 1945. A significant number of Krios emigrated, and by applying their talents and skills made contributions to the development of other areas of West Africa, ranging from the Gambia to the Congo.

THE SOCIETY OF THE INTERIOR

While the culture of the Krios dominated Freetown and the peninsula region - the area of the original colony - and flourished well into the twentieth century, the interior of the country experienced a different kind of development. In effect, two societies evolved. One became urban and cosmopolitan, integrating, but not rejecting, the African past and culture with the Western world; the other society remained rural, traditional, and tribalized.

At the very beginning of the colony, in the late eighteenth century, trading contacts existed between Freetown and the interior. By that time, numerous ethnic groups had settled and controlled areas of the hinterland. Some of these included the Limba, the oldest one, along with the Soso or Susu, the Vai and Kono, the Koranko, the Kissi, the Yalunka, the Loko, and the Sherbro.[2] The Mende and the Temne dominated sizeable areas and became the two largest ethnic groups.

While each culture was unique, these nineteenth century tribal states did share certain common characteristics: war accounted for the origins of most of the states, and the size and power of each one was determined largely by the fortunes of combat. A king stood at the top of society; the Temne called him O'bai, the Mende named him Mahin. He dispensed justice, and often was both a prominent trader and a skilled warrior. His state embraced villages and towns, collected into districts, with each subdivision under a local ruler or chief. A group of elders formed a council to assist the king; they were old men who, along with other aged members of society, received and enjoyed the respect of the community, particularly the young.

Most people were small farmers, living together in a household, better known in Sierra Leone as a compound. It comprised a person's extended family and was the basic unit of farming; members of the compound worked as a unit in the fields, sowing the seeds and harvesting the crops.

Secret societies, a constant in West African cultures, offered social and educational outlets, chiefly for the young. Restricted to members of the same gender in a specific area of the country, the societies conducted private activities in secluded settings, keeping out aliens and strangers. The Poro, a male society, and the Bundo, a female society, were the important ones. The Bundo trained girls for womanhood, teaching such areas of domestic science as child care and hygiene. The Poro, on the other hand, was intensely political. Its oaths of secrecy were strictly observed and enforced. Along with initiating boys into manhood and offering training in fighting and hunting, its leadership made decisions regarding such important matters as war and the harvesting of valuable crops.

Along with the prevalence of secret societies, religion permeated the cultures of the interior. Residents of the tribal states believed in several gods, with one much more important than the others: the Temne named him Kru, the Mende, Ngewoh. Both Christianity and Islam spread into the interior. Only a few Christian missions existed; Islam received a larger following, mainly because it adapted easily to such traditional customs as polygamy.

After mid-century, a well-established and thriving trade network existed between Freetown and the interior. In trying to control or acquire a share of this prosperous activity, the tribal states competed and frequently fought petty wars. These conflicts disrupted commerce and stirred demands for British intervention. Some influential Krios in Freetown called for the annexation of more territory to the colony. The colonial administration did make some ineffectual moves to assure peace and stability over the trade routes. British policy, however, remained vague until challenged by the threat of French intervention.

With control over Guinea, the area to the north and east of Sierra Leone, the French stood in a commanding position to manipulate events in the hinterland. Tribal unrest had in fact brought French arms to the interior, an alarming development for the administration in Freetown. At this time, the last decade of the nineteenth century, the British and the French were competing fiercely for spheres of influence throughout the world. The tense atmosphere between the two powers could escalate any minor incident into a major crisis. This situation was averted in West Africa, however. England and France signed an agreement delineating the territory to each power. Soon after, in 1898, a British protectorate was proclaimed in Sierra Leone, uniting the colony, that is Freetown and the peninsula area, with the interior. Hereafter both geographical regions were identified as Sierra Leone.

This union between colony and protectorate remained superficial for some time. Colonial policy continually worked against fusion of the two cultures. For example, the British decision to help finance the administration of the newly declared protectorate

by means of a tax levy on the huts or houses of the interior produced resistance and rebellion, a series of events best known as
the Hut Tax War of 1898. There were revolts throughout the protectorate, and in some areas ugly incidents occurred. Property
was destroyed and persons identified with aliens or the British,
notably Krios, were indiscriminately attacked or killed. Such
events left a legacy of bad feelings between Krios and other
peoples of the interior; in a broader context, the Hut Tax War
reflected the inadequacies of colonial policy that, in effect, had
created a division between colony and protectorate.

The opening decades of the twentieth century witnessed the
emergence of a new social order in Sierra Leone. Its most obvious feature was the diminution of Krio power and influence, a
result of late-nineteenth century policy of discrimination by the
colonial government. For example, appointments to senior positions in the administration now went to Europeans rather than
Krios, and when a Krio official retired or died, a European replaced him. Over time, with the implementation of this policy,
the position of the Krios in the colonial hierarchy weakened significantly. Krio medical doctors met the same kind of intolerance.

A new group of migrants, the Lebanese or Syrians, entering
West Africa in the 1890s, proved themselves skilled in trade.
They offered forceful competition to Krio business, and rose
rapidly to play a significant role in the economy. The rise of an
indigenous protectorate elite also undercut Krio influence. This
was a slowly developing process, chiefly because of the lack of
adequate educational facilities in the interior. Most of the educated individuals in the protectorate received a higher education
at Fourah Bay College, but large numbers of trained professionals did not emerge from the protectorate until after World
War II. At that time, a most auspicious period for Sierra Leone,
the country was on the eve of emancipation from colonial rule,
and the new protectorate elite stood in a position to exert a powerful influence over the independence movement.

TOWARD INDEPENDENCE - AND BEYOND

British authorities adapted to the drive for independence.
Emerging from World War II as an exhausted and weakened
power, Britain faced demands from people all over the empire
who wanted more autonomy from the mother country. In West

Africa, where the British had acted more as temporary residents than permanent settlers, the transition from colony to nation was logical and orderly, a matter largely of timing and tactics. The course for independence in Sierra Leone was set by constitutional practice and emerging representative institutions. New constitutional proposals were introduced in 1947 that were to expand the representation of the protectorate in the Legislative Council, a small deliberative body created in 1863 and enlarged slightly in 1924. This change would give a majority to the protectorate members of the council, a development that alarmed many Krios, who feared protectorate domination. They tried unsuccessfully to prevent the adoption of the 1947 proposals.

This divisiveness faded. By the mid-1950s, the spokespeople of the protectorate - the educated elite as well as the traditional authorities - along with some Krios from the colony, had come together in the Sierra Leone Peoples Party (SLPP). Other developments reflected unity and movement toward independence. More Africans assumed responsibility for ministries in the government; universal adult suffrage was introduced; the Legislative Council became larger and was renamed the House of Representatives.

There was dissent within the SLPP, coming largely from younger members who wanted more African control over the government and a faster timetable for independence. This protest was contained by bringing together leading politicians into a United National Front to work for independence. A constitutional convention met in London to work out the transfer of power agreements. Soon after, on April 27, 1961, the anniversary date of the Mende uprising against the Hut Tax in 1898, Sierra Leone became an independent nation-state.

After independence, a strong opposition party emerged, the All Peoples Congress (APC). The APC captured popularity and support, diminishing the prestige and power of the SLPP. The appeal of the SLPP was weakened by a slipping economy and the party's identification with unpopular issues and corruption. Elections called in 1967 gave a majority to the APC. The military would not accept the results, and an army coup ensued, forcing the APC leadership into exile; power then passed to a National Reformation Council (NRC), a group of army officers and police officers. Within a year, revulsion against the corruption in the NRC and dissatisfaction among young army officers led to another army coup. This time the military called for a return to civilian rule. The APC leaders, notably Siaka Stevens, were invited back from exile to form a new government. Parliamentary rule was restored.

Dissatisfaction, however, remained profound and widespread. Charges of corruption and dictatorship became commonplace between opposing factions; violent confrontations occurred, and there were more attempts to overthrow the government. In facing these events, the Stevens administration took a firm position and ignored constitutional proprieties. It gave much publicity to the trial and execution of the leaders of a disaffected APC group who had attempted a coup. Still, tranquillity remained elusive. Fighting occurred in the Pujehun District, and many refugees went to Liberia. Student demonstrations increased, threatening public order.

During these years of tension and instability, Sierra Leone became a republic (1971) and a one-party state (1978). The APC maintained control over the government and successfully transferred power in the mid-1980s. Siaka Stevens stepped down and on January 26, 1986, was replaced by Joseph Momoh. This smooth succession was an important precedent and stabilizing factor for the political system of Sierra Leone.

ECONOMIC DEVELOPMENTS

The most fundamental issue facing the Momoh administration was the critical, deteriorating state of the economy, an enduring problem for Sierra Leone.[3] Before independence, during the 1950s, the country experienced general prosperity. The mining of iron ore and diamonds accounted largely for the economic good times. Iron deposits at Marampa in northern Sierra Leone yielded high-grade ore, attracting overseas interests and markets. The Sierra Leone Development Company (DELCO) acquired exclusive rights from the colonial government to extract ore, and it constructed a railroad, connecting the ore fields to port facilities at Pepel.

Diamonds were first discovered in the Kenema and Kono districts of eastern Sierra Leone. Again, the government entrusted a company, the Sierra Leone Selection Trust (SLST), with a monopoly to mine diamonds. In return, SLST, like DELCO, made payments to the government; the company, in effect, gave a share of its profits to the state. Both SLST and DELCO began mining in the 1930s, and by the 1950s each was engaged in large-scale operations.

Many problems came from the mine fields. Initially, mining diamonds did not require the expensive, heavy earth-moving equipment needed for extracting iron ore. Diamonds could be found by using pans to wash gravel in river beds. After World War II, a diamond rush occurred: thousands of people, driven by visions of acquiring great wealth, descended into the area. This migration disrupted traditional agricultural labor and authority. Many people abandoned chores and responsibilities, and ignored paternalistic advice.

By the 1950s, between 50,000 and 70,000 people were searching for diamonds in eastern Sierra Leone. A few found riches, most did not, and lived in squalor, digging and fantasizing about gaining a quick fortune. All of this illegal activity could not be controlled, forcing the government to make a new agreement with SLST. The trust narrowed its area of monopoly to approximately 500 square miles, and individuals were permitted to mine legally after securing a license from the government. Still, illicit mining occurred, and the smuggling of diamonds remained a serious, unresolvable problem.

Throughout the 1950s, and well into the 1960s, the exploitation of the country's mineral wealth brought in revenue and encouraged development. In 1950, mining revenue was around three million pounds; in 1958, the amount was over ten million pounds. Now the government could spend money on needed services and projects. New educational, medical, and welfare services and facilities were established. Secondary education expanded. Fourah Bay College was relocated on a new campus laid out on Mount Aureol high above Freetown. Numerous projects were introduced to facilitate trade and travel: internal air transport was started, a new international airport was constructed at Lungi, steel bridges replaced ferries across rivers, many roads were built, and a deep-water quay was completed in Freetown. All of these varied activities and projects fostered economic well-being and facilitated Sierra Leone's transition from colony to independent state.

Prosperity began ebbing in the late 1960s; over the years, the economy floundered and followed a descending course. The economy remained sluggish and underdeveloped in the early 1990s. Both internal and external factors contributed to Sierra Leone's economic malaise. Basic to the economic downturn was the apparent dwindling of mineral wealth. The annual output of diamonds and iron ore dropped sharply. Local diamond exports, for example, stood around two million carats in 1970; this amount had fallen to approximately 303,000 in 1982. With diamonds accounting for over 50 percent of the country's export earnings, this steep decline had a crippling effect on the economy.

An effort to reverse the trend came in August 1984 with the creation of the Precious Minerals Marketing Company. Owned by the government and local diamond dealers, it aimed at maintaining market prices and fighting smugglers. A proposal for deep underground mining also raised hope for Sierra Leone diamond production. Financing for this project, however, has remained elusive; and the factors causing the decrease in diamond exports have endured, notably the depletion of accessible deposits, the drop in international diamond prices, and most important, an intensification of smuggling.

Iron ore was the second most important mineral export until the early 1970s, when production sunk. The Marampa mines were forced to close in 1975, all the ore apparently removed and exported. Continued effort and concern, along with an Austrian loan, facilitated the reopening of the mines in 1983. Ore shipments resumed, but never reached previous high levels, and were often interrupted by labor disturbances. In contrast to the downtrend in diamond and iron ore production, exports of bauxite and rutile have increased - a positive, though limited, economic development.

Throughout the 1980s, the manufacturing sector of the economy, which accounted for only 5 percent of the gross national product, declined. The shortage of foreign exchange caused this retarded industrial output. The most important manufactured goods were tobacco, liquor, matches, nails, and various food products. In addition, agriculture, the largest sector of the economy, was depressed; it employed about 70 percent of the work force, primarily at the subsistence level. Only 30 percent of agricultural production was available for marketing. The most important agricultural exports were coffee, cocoa, and palm kernels, each one vulnerable to the fluctuating prices of the world market. The dismal state of agriculture in Sierra Leone was reflected in the fact that rice, the staple of the local diet, had to be imported in large quantities to feed the population.

The economic difficulties of the country have been aggravated, or perhaps caused, by government policies, a condition most evident from the late 1970s onward. The government has consistently failed to collect all revenues and to control expenditures. An obvious manifestation of this failure of policy has been the budget deficits, a constant in recent administrative history. Often budgets have increased several times during a fiscal year. The government was unable to combat or even check the deterioration of the economy. This situation left the system vulnerable to charges of corruption. It discouraged foreign investments and alarmed international creditors. Within Sierra Leone, it generated cynicism and resentment.

Throughout the 1980s, the government experienced a series of economic crises, many characterized by severe shortages of petroleum and rice. Inflation plagued the country: in the late 1970s, inflation averaged 15 percent annually; it rose steadily from 11 to 31 percent from 1980 to 1982; in 1983, consumer prices in Freetown increased by over 78 percent. Power outages occurred daily. To be sure, the high price of oil was an important factor upsetting the economy and unbalancing budgets. Still, an inept administration, coupled with mistaken policies, created much distress. Sharp criticism persisted for years over the large sums of money spent by the government to host the Organization of African Unity (OAU) conference in Freetown in June 1980.

The basic economic fact of the country remains: most Sierra Leoneans live at a subsistence level - they cannot afford to purchase nonessential goods. A family's income is spent on the basic items of survival, that is, food, housing, transportation, and clothing. When economic conditions worsen, a higher percentage of income must go to food. Often, there are difficulties acquiring such basic commodities as gasoline, kerosene, and rice. Under such conditions, living is hazardous, causing much physical and emotional stress, along with marital and family discord.

CULTURAL TRAITS

These harsh circumstances are sustained and rationalized by a deterministic outlook on life, which views the status quo as the only reality. Any change or alternative to existing conditions cannot be imagined. In other words, in Sierra Leone, deprivation is accepted as the norm. The psychological corollary to this outlook is the practice of denial. The problems of life are evaded by refusing to admit that any exist. This stance is accompanied by a carefree attitude. People do complain, and criticize, and make sharp comments about misspent money, the petrol shortages, and the corruption of businessmen and government officials. But there is little bitterness, no rancor, and life continues with apparent enjoyment; people remain easygoing. Among important social groups, parties begin at 11:00 p.m. and continue unabated until 6:00 a.m. An often-heard remark is that "Africa" is to blame for any trouble or inconvenience. Getting caught without warning or apparent reason, for example, in an inextricable traffic jam, elicits the expression "Africa," implying that the incident typifies the unpredictable and frustrating way of life in the Third World.

This conviviality, acting as a defense mechanism to gloss over the harsher side of life, forms part of the normality threshold in Sierra Leone society. A reserved demeanor represents another important quality; people frown on using offensive language and disapprove of loud, boisterous behavior. Any kind of violent conduct is condemned. And special value is attached to maintaining one's respect for elders, a strongly held belief that extends to strangers. A young man, for example, may view an older man with the same high regard as he holds for his father.

In this society, individualism is contained, never exalted. The driving personality so common to industrial societies has no place in West Africa. While a person's capacity to make choices and assume responsibilities remains an essential and admirable trait, much of Sierra Leonean life carries a group rather than an individual orientation. The ethnic group, the village, and the family form extended networks of cohesion and identity for the individual. No one is alone or alienated or outside of the mainstream of life. A chain of groups sustain and restrain the individual.

This predominance of the group over the individual shields and offers support for a person who, from a European perspective, might be labeled a moral transgressor or a deviant. In many Western societies, for example, an unmarried woman who has a baby is stigmatized and isolated; she and the child become moral outcasts, her offspring designated illegitimate, to be kept beyond the pale of respectable society.

In contrast, a woman in Sierra Leone who has a child out of wedlock finds that both she and the infant are accepted into the family. The father of the baby is known; he receives little pressure to marry but is encouraged to provide some kind of child support. A compelling need encourages a woman, whether single or married, to have a child: the child will care for the mother in her old age. A woman is reproached, then, if she has no children. While not ostracized, a barren woman arouses concern, suspicion, and disdain; prevailing sentiment assumes that something must be wrong with her. Some form of witchcraft, frequently, is held accountable for her condition.

A deviant individual, such as a mentally ill person, is also kept within a strong web of groups. The extended family accepts the responsibility for the care of their mentally distressed kin, and some family member will attend to the needs of the sick person. Leaders of the patient's ethnic and religious groups provide additional support, offering prayers and ceremonies, further protecting the disturbed individual from social isolation.

This informal network of associations breaks down, however, when the mentally disordered person becomes violent. Anyone exhibiting bizarre and assaultive behavior poses a problem, and institutionalization, either with a traditional healer or at a psychiatric facility, is viewed as the best way of handling such a threat to the community.

In contrast, the nonmenacing, eccentric mentally ill are tolerated and roam freely about the streets. There are numerous examples. For instance, a slender middle-aged woman, who usually carries a large bundle of sticks on her head, stands across the street from the administration building on the campus of Fourah Bay College and babbles for several minutes. She claims ownership of all the property and buildings on campus. While she makes a fuss, people walk by, giving her scant attention. Eventually she leaves, only to return a few days or weeks later to continue her diatribe.

In another recently observed case, an ex-mental patient, a man about 30 years old, camps out near the Cotton Tree in downtown Freetown. The tree, over 200 years old, is one of the country's most important landmarks and stands in the middle of the busiest traffic circle of the city. It has a huge trunk with several large crevices, and this man lives in one that he has screened off with a stiff bamboo curtain. Most of the time he sleeps on the ground, or sits and watches the traffic. On occasion, he will pace about the tree in his underwear, breathing heavily. He is left alone, unless detained by the authorities who think that tourists might see him and take offense.

In another instance, a middle-aged man, an ex-mental patient, stages a "crazy" public performance, acting out the role of a madman. On a busy street, he will grimace, gesticulate, dance, and move about in a wild nonsensical manner, to the amusement and fascination of a gathering crowd. Some onlookers pass coins to him, appreciating the show.

The tolerance extended to these and other odd but nonviolent mentally ill persons may reflect the open, diverse character of Freetown. In Western cities, the police quickly neutralize any kind of disturbance or challenge to order and to the flow of traffic. In African cities, people, rather than traffic, dominate the streets. Rich and poor, foreigner and native, beggar and merchant rub shoulders and interact - trading, bargaining, cajoling, exchanging greetings and insults. In this busy cosmopolitan atmosphere, a person acting in an unusual but nonthreatening manner may be watched or ignored, but rarely is restrained or harmed by strangers or authorities.

The cause of bizarre conduct, however, excites concern and generates apprehension. The toleration given to the public behavior of deviant or mentally ill people, coupled with the integration of such individuals in a strong web of groups, may militate against individual anomie. This fact obscures a preoccupation with the meaning and relief of human misfortune. Any kind of trouble stirs anxieties, encouraging speculation about its true nature and significance.

Such concern touches everyday mundane affairs. The inscriptions on lorries represent one of its manifestations. Lorries are decorated with mottoes, epigrams, and sayings, painted in bold colors on the vehicles. Each inscription, written in Krio, reveals the attitudes or preoccupations of the lorry driver. Many of these sayings express feelings of insecurity and anxiety; others reveal a paranoid fear that someone or something, envious and malevolent, will inflict great harm on the vehicle owner.

The sayings represent a way of neutralizing or fighting back at the malefactor; more important, they reflect the broader cultural preoccupation, pervasive throughout the society, of attributing the source of human adversity to powerful, unseen, supernatural forces bent on humbling and controlling the individual.

NOTES

1. This brief historical survey is based largely on the following sources: Christopher Fyfe, *A History of Sierra Leone* (London: Oxford University Press, 1962); Christopher Fyfe, *A Short History of Sierra Leone* (London: Longman, 1979); C. Magbaily Fyle, *The History of Sierra Leone* (London: Evans Brothers, 1981); Leo Spitzer, *The Creoles of Sierra Leone: Responses to Colonialism, 1870-1945* (Madison: University of Wisconsin Press, 1974); Akintola J. G. Wyse, "Some Thoughts on Sierra Leone History," *Journal of the Historical Society of Sierra Leone* 2 (Jan. 1978): 1-9; A.J.G. Wyse, *Searchlight on the Krio of Sierra Leone: An Ethnographical Study of a West Af-*

rican People, Occasional Paper no. 3, Institute of African Studies, Fourah Bay College, 1980; Akintola Wyse,*The Krio of Sierra Leone: An Interpretive History* (Freetown: Okrafo-Smart, 1989); Abner Cohen, *The Politics of Elite Culture: Explorations in the Dramaturgy of Power in a Modern African Society* (Berkeley: University of California Press, 1981); H. L. van der Laan, *The Lebanese Traders in Sierra Leone* (The Hague 1975); Neil O. Leighton, "The Political Economy of a Stranger Population: The Lebanese of Sierra Leone," in William A. Shack and Elliott P. Skinner, eds., *Strangers in African Societies* (Berkeley: University of California Press, 1979), 85-103; Cyril P. Foray, *Historical Dictionary of Sierra Leone* (Metuchen, N.J.: Scarecrow Press, 1977); Martin Kilson, *Political Change in a West African State: A Study of the Modernization Process in Sierra Leone* (New York: Antheum, 1969); Murray Last, Paul Richards, and Christopher Fyfe, eds., *Sierra Leone 1787-1987: Two Centuries of Intellectual Life* (Manchester: Manchester University Press, 1987); Christopher Fyfe and Eldred Jones, *Freetown: A Symposium* (Freetown: Sierra Leone University Press, 1968); and Joe A. D. Alie, *A New History of Sierra Leone* (New York: St. Martin's Press, 1990).

2. The spelling of ethnic designations varies among authors and among published and unpublished sources. Throughout this study, the author tried to remain consistent, but did make compromises between historical and contemporary preferences. For example, while "Krio" rather than "Creole" was used in most instances, such spellings as "Foulah" and "Susu" and "Kroo" were observed rather than "Fula" or "Soso" or "Kru." The rationale for using a particular spelling related to its popular or preferred spelling, as well as its continued appearance in the written sources.

3. The major sources used for this survey of the economy of Sierra Leone include: "Sierra Leone," in *Africa South of the Sahara 1984-85* (London: Europa Publications, 1984), 744-58; *Sierra Leone, Country Plan* (United States Information Agency, Freetown, Sierra Leone, 1986); *Foreign Economic Trends and Their Implications for the United States, Sierra Leone*, prepared by the American Embassy, Freetown (U.S. Department of Commerce, April 1985); Fyfe, *A Short History of Sierra Leone*, 143, 146-48, 156-57; Fyle, *The History of Sierra Leone*, 130-36, 143-44; and H. L. van der Laan, *The Sierra Leone Diamonds: An Economic Study Covering the Years 1952-1961* (London: Oxford University Press, 1965).

3 The Institution

Throughout most of the nineteenth century, Kissy Lunatic Asylum in Sierra Leone was the only agency of Western mental health care in British West Africa. This institution grew slowly and took time to develop a clear identity; for many years, it functioned largely as a place of detention for varied kinds of dependents. In the first half of the nineteenth century, the medical services of the colony remained quite limited. The authorities were preoccupied with such public health concerns as sanitation and sewage disposal, as well as the high mortality rate of Europeans living and working in West Africa. By the 1870s, solutions to these problems were evolving and a network of medical services and facilities existed. The asylum was recognized solely as a mental institution, a separate and necessary part of the colonial medical system. Over time, it acquired the status of a mental hospital and gradually adopted the therapeutics of Western psychiatric facilities.

Early in the history of the colony, health matters aroused special interest. On the crowded slave ships, disease broke out and spread rapidly. Epidemics of ophthalmia, dysentery, and smallpox were common. Some recaptives arrived sick, requiring immediate medical attention and treatment. In 1817, concerned about the physical and mental condition of the recaptives, the colonial government established a hospital in Freetown. The entrance gate still stands as a historic landmark, and it carries an inscription that captures the purpose and spirit of the early colony. Embedded in the stone arch over the gate are the words: "Royal Hospital and Asylum for Africans Rescued from Slavery by British Valour and Philanthropy."

In actual practice, this facility functioned initially as a medical triage office. The sick went to Regent, a community a few miles to the southeast, or to a recaptive hospital, which operated out of a missionary building in Leicester, a village near Regent, high up in mountains above Freetown. In other places, local networks provided care. Benevolent societies, for example, attended to their sick members and buried those who died. Some mad people were kept in the Freetown Gaol.[1]

Beginning in the mid-1820s, and continuing throughout the next decade, a building located in the village of Kissy, a community northeast of Freetown, attached to the Liberated African Department of the colonial government, became the depository for groups of undifferentiated dependents, including the sick, the aged, and the insane. In 1844, this facility was designated a colonial hospital. It received the sick poor, invalid recaptives, and destitute European sailors, as well as lunatics sent from the Freetown Gaol. Nearby, a lazaretto housed smallpox patients.[2]

Almost from the onset, the colonial hospital at Kissy lacked direction and was burdened by mismanagement. Living conditions deteriorated, the result of a lax, inefficient, and indifferent administration. Patients were herded into dirty wards; they slept on floor mats and were maintained on inadequate rations. The institution had no direct medical supervision. By the late 1840s, it served around 400 patients suffering from varied physical and mental disorders, but by that time there was a resident physician. This fact, coupled with the increasing number of patients and the decaying physical condition of the facility, led the colonial government, in 1851, to transfer the hospital to Queen's Yard in Freetown. Only lunatics, incurables, and smallpox patients remained at the Kissy institution, and each group was kept apart from the others.[3]

COLONIAL HEALTH CONCERNS

By the mid-nineteenth century, sanitation and related health problems in Freetown could not be overlooked, and finally aroused government concern and attention. The city had experienced rapid growth which strained facilities and created unhygienic conditions. Piles of decaying vegetation and garbage polluted the streets; open cesspits, close to houses, functioned as privies and contained heaps of decomposing excreta. Observers noted that these conditions, combined with the sun's heat, produced "unhealthy vapors" that formed a misty cloud hovering over the city.

Such comments reflected the prevailing miasma theory of disease. Miasma was described as "thick air," "dangerous dampness of air," "noxious gas," or "offending harmful gases." Mid-nineteenth century medical opinion identified miasma as the cause of tropical fevers; it was thought to originate from varied sources, including swamps, rotting ships, and bilge water. However, a combination of decay, particularly of vegetable matter, heat, and dampness constituted its basic genesis. The search for sources of miasma fostered the field of medical topography, which became a major preoccupation of British medical men in West Africa. Many of these physicians published the results of their observations and findings; a few offered solutions.

James Boyle, an acting colonial surgeon in Sierra Leone, went beyond compiling data and proposed a scheme to protect Freetown from nearby swamps. He suggested draining the area, keeping it clear of bush, and, during the wet season, burning continuous fires in clay kilns. The carbon dioxide from the fires would purify the air before it reached Freetown. A few years later, another plan, presented by F. Harrison Ranklin, focused on the same area, the swampland across the Sierra Leone River from Freetown. Ranklin's plan called for the construction of a wall thirty feet high and eighteen miles long. The structure would protect the city from the "travelling miasma," an assumed deadly substance that clung close to the ground.[4]

While these schemes were not implemented, colonial administrators remained sensitive to assumptions about the sources of miasma and urged people to be attentive to sanitation. Some public latrines and baths were constructed in Freetown. In the early 1870s, Governor John Pope Hennessy employed a corps of sweepers and scavengers to clean the city. This group collected dead animals, chiefly dogs, hogs, and goats, off the streets; it inspected open springs and water courses; it cleared streets of rubbish and filth. Hennessy remained so disturbed by Freetown's unsanitary conditions that he called for the removal of the entire government to the mountains. This project was rejected; still, sick English people often moved to mountain areas to recuperate from fever illnesses, thinking that the higher altitude protected them from threatening miasmic vapors.[5]

Throughout the second half of the nineteenth century, colonial administrators were perplexed and alarmed by health problems that related more to Europeans than Africans. For Europeans, the danger of being stricken by some fatal disease represented a silent but constant threat: living in Sierra Leone carried a much greater risk than residing in Europe. Insurance companies refused to extend a policy to anyone going to Freetown. A haunting image of death enveloped Sierra Leone, designating it as "the white man's grave."

The high mortality rate was initially attributed to such traditional factors as climate, bad air from swamps, and the imbalance of bodily fluids. When more precise scientific knowledge was applied to tropical health problems, toward the end of the century, malaria and yellow fever were identified as the killer diseases. In the late 1890s, Richard Ross, a lecturer at the Liverpool School of Tropical Medicine, specified the mosquito as the vector for malaria, and actually spent time in Sierra Leone confirming the results of his research. Working also in the tropics, notably in the East Indies as well as in Africa, Richard Koch, a German scientist, corroborated the effectiveness of quinine as a method of containing the disease.

Along with eliminating the breeding grounds of mosquitoes and inaugurating mass quininization programs, some malariologists stressed another preventive measure: segregating Europeans from Africans. Here the argument centered on the presumed attraction of mosquitoes to Africans. If these insects were indeed drawn to Africans, and hovered about their settlements, a logical conclusion followed: the health of Europeans would be enhanced by being removed from the source of attraction.

On the basis of this assumption, coupled with cultural and racial arrogance, beliefs about contagion, plus the long-standing interest in moving to higher elevations, colonial administrators in Sierra Leone developed an exclusive residential area above Freetown. Called Hill Station, it was segregated completely from the African community.[6]

Some Krios criticized the expenditure for Hill Station, noting that the government spent only trifling sums on improvements in Freetown.[7] This was a valid point. Throughout the late nineteenth century, the financial situation of the colony remained serious. The Colonial Office in London often urged governors of Sierra Leone to cut expenses and operate on a minimal budget. With limited funds available, they stipulated that only absolutely necessary repairs on streets and buildings be made; expanding or undertaking new social services was not possible.[8]

All of the interest and concern devoted to understanding and combatting malaria and yellow fever obscured the problems associated with other tropical diseases. While malaria remained endemic throughout the country, causing much ill-health and producing a high mortality rate among African children, many other diseases tormented Africans more than Europeans. Sierra Leone could not be designated a grave for any special race; it was everyone's grave. The health condition of Africans remained poor. Few nineteenth century European physicians took interest in Guinea worm, yaws, leprosy, elephantiasis, trypanosomiasis, and other diseases that struck chiefly Africans.[9]

Trypanosomiasis, a fatal paralytic disease, came into Sierra Leone with the tsetse fly during the middle decades of the nineteenth century after the tall forests had been cut down. This insect bites horses and cattle, infecting them with the disease. It cannot breed in high forests but requires shade close to the ground. Along the coastal regions, with the timber cut and exported, a favorable environment was created for the tsetse fly.[10] Trypanosomiasis also affected humans, and became popularly known as sleeping sickness; many afflicted with the disease displayed unusual behavior and were sent to the lunatic asylum for observation and treatment.

THE ORGANIZATION AND REGIMEN OF THE ASYLUM

By the 1870s, the Kissy institution for the insane was one of several facilities operated by the medical department of the colonial government of Sierra Leone. The prime institution was the Colonial Hospital in Freetown; other facilities included the Gaol Hospital, the Colonial Hospital at Sherbro, and three District Dispensaries. At Kissy, the Smallpox Hospital and the Hospital for Incurables were located near the lunatic asylum. The Hospital for Incurables cared for Africans with incurable diseases as well as the old, the infirm, and persons without a means of livelihood.

All of these facilities were administered by the colonial surgeon, the most important and highest-ranking medical officer in the country. The colonial surgeon reported directly to the governor of the colony. While assigned to manage the institutions "for the humane care of patients," his many assignments and obligations limited his direct involvement in the daily functioning of each facility.

A resident superintendent, for example, directed the affairs of the lunatic asylum. His responsibilities included maintaining order and discipline, instructing the staff, controlling food rations, regulating inventories, and dispensing drugs and medicine. Always on call, he was never to be away from the asylum for more than two hours a day. In the late nineteenth century, the resident superintendency often remained vacant because of the shortage of medical doctors in the colony. In actual practice, then, a lay keeper, who lived on the premises, supervised day-to-day operations. A medical officer, a physician from the staff of the colonial surgeon, paid weekly and, on occasion, semiweekly visits to Kissy.[11]

The asylum existed solely for the care of "the insane and the idiotic," with admissions and discharges controlled by the written approval of the chief justice of the colonial government. There was an additional check: before being admitted, or discharged, a patient had to be certified insane, or sane, by "two properly qualified medical men." A board of inspection, appointed by the governor, functioned as a watchdog committee to maintain standards and prevent abuses. It reported on asylum conditions twice a year. The board members remained most attentive to maintenance problems and patient requests and complaints. An 1887 report lamented the poor physical condition of the institution and noted that the patients had no complaints, "but many of them asked to be allowed to go home."[12]

A strict regimen governed institutional life. The sexes were separated. During the day, patients remained in their respective enclosures and yards, "always under the eyes of the keeper and the attendants." Breakfast was served at nine, dinner at four. At night, between six and six, patients were locked in dormitories. An attendant slept in the male ward, a nurse in the female quarters. At all times, the institution was physically locked from the outside community. A guard secured the front gate, and no person entered or left the asylum without the knowledge of the keeper or the medical officer. Those entering or leaving signed a gatebook, a record of daily traffic. Other important matters were carefully recorded: a register of admissions listed the names of patients admitted for treatment; a medical case book noted the progress or retrogression of each inmate; a daily medical journal recorded all prescriptions ordered for the use of patients. Inspectors scrutinized these books, picking at random a name off the register of admission, for example, and calling for the certificate of insanity that authorized that patient's detention in the asylum.[13]

Kindness was proclaimed as the guiding principle of care. A policy of nonrestraint prevailed, and coercive measures were utilized only in cases of violence or attempted escapes. No specific type of therapy was advocated. Work was encouraged, but only among the "more intelligent and docile" patients, who performed such casual labor as gardening, carrying water, cleaning, and sweeping. Some inmates made straw hats and repaired clothing. The administration also encouraged patients to amuse themselves with games and dances. A pleasant diversion occurred on holidays, namely Christmas and Easter, when religious groups and community residents gave presents of fruit, ginger beer, tobacco, and biscuits to the patients.[14]

BASIC PROBLEMS

Throughout the late nineteenth century, some fundamental problems preoccupied asylum administrators. Overcrowded burial grounds produced embarrassment when a grave-digging detail, composed of laborers and patients, struck human remains.[15] But the need for a new, larger cemetery was obscured by a more pressing concern: establishing a better way of supplying water. The staff, and, at times, the patients, drew water from a nearby stream and carried it several hundred yards to the asylum. During the dry season, this became a painfully slow, inefficient, and inadequate operation.[16]

Another fundamental problem was simply the task of maintaining the institution. The asylum needed repairs and renovation. A number of administrative reports and inspections referred to the physical plant as "defective" or "in a very unsatisfactory state"; the 1892 annual report of the medical department called for the building of a new lunatic asylum, noting that "the present buildings, dormitories, and single cells are of obsolete pattern."[17]

Many factors contributed to the decay of facilities: the old age of the structures, wood-eating ants, violent weather, particularly lightning storms, and the destruction caused by violent patients. Requisitions for immediate repairs remained a constant; the usual demands called for changing shutters, lime-washing floors and walls, rehanging windows, stopping roof leaks, and replacing locks, hinges, doors, windows, and floor joists and joints.[18]

The dilapidated physical condition of some areas of the asylum encouraged patients to run away. This situation led the colonial surgeon to write to the governor, informing him that the rash of recent escapes was "in consequence of the insecure conditions of the institution from want of repairs." Many doors and windows needed replacement; such repairs were essential "for the safe keeping of these dangerous persons." The plea did not win the support of the governor. Requisitions for repairs to the lunatic asylum were denied, "for want of funds."[19]

Many escapes could not be attributed to the run-down physical condition of the institution. Staff negligence also played a role. Those who allowed a patient to escape were punished. For example, after a female patient who broke out of the asylum was found and brought back, the assistant female warden was "fined five shillings as it was through her carelessness that the lunatic escaped."[20] In another case, an attendant was fined for failing to lock a gate through which a patient escaped.[21] When a patient ran away from a work detail that was collecting sticks and stones outside of the asylum, the supervising attendant was dismissed.[22] The fining or dismissal of negligent or incompetent staff occurred frequently, and, in some instances, lengthy, detailed investigations occurred. Clearly, the medical authorities in Freetown believed that the escape of any mental patient from Kissy was a serious matter.[23]

Despite difficulties with the buildings and staff, the admission and discharge of patients was carefully monitored. In most instances, legal and medical regulations made the acceptance and release of inmates a routine, orderly manner. Regarding admission, a certificate of lunacy authorized the detention of a person, citing the reason for confinement. A court order followed, and a medical examination, administered by two physicians, took place. If found mad, the individual was declared "a lunatic, and a proper person to be confined in the Lunatic Asylum."[24] A discharge reversed this process. As with the admission procedure, often a relative initiated the action. At the asylum, a physician reported on the patient's condition. If that recommendation was favorable, a higher medical and legal authority reviewed the case, and, finding no irregularities, certified the individual sane and determined the time of release.[25]

There were cases that required special attention and consideration. Admissions and discharges were sometimes denied. For example, a son wanted his mother placed in the asylum, arguing that she was in a "wretched and miserable state" and used obscene language in public. After observing her for a few days in the Colonial Hospital in Freetown, medical authorities reported that "we can find no trace of lunacy sufficient to send her to the Lunatic Asylum at Kissy."[26] In another case, a man demanded that his brother be admitted to the asylum because he was "an extremely dangerous character." Observing physicians, however, found no reason for confining the man.[27]

A request for an inmate's discharge was always denied if the patient posed a threat to the community. A man's plea for his son's release was turned down because the son was "insane and violent" and frequently had to be kept isolated in a confinement cell.[28] A sister of a male patient requested her brother's discharge, claiming that a native healer in Freetown could cure him. The colonial surgeon rejected the demand, pointing out that her brother "is a dangerous lunatic and unfit to be at large."[29]

On the other hand, a plea for the dismissal of a well-behaved, rational patient, sponsored by a responsible person, received quick attention and approval. A woman suffering from "alcoholic mania" remained in the asylum for a week; each day her condition improved. Her daughter applied for the mother's discharge, promising that she would go "to the rivers for native treatment." The colonial surgeon consented, specifying the condition that the mother actually receive native care.[30] In another instance, a Liberian woman petitioned the governor of Sierra Leone for the removal of her son from Kissy so that he might return home with her to Liberia. He had been an inmate for over three years. An asylum report disclosed that the son "has been a quiet patient, speaks very little, and is always willing to do any work." At times he "becomes wild," but never dangerous. After the governor determined, through Liberian authorities, the trustworthiness of the woman, the patient was released to her custody.[31]

CHARACTERISTICS OF PATIENTS

Insane criminals or prisoners made up a segment of the asylum clientele that required particular scrutiny. Some criminals never went to prison; they were convicted, certified insane, and sent directly to Kissy. For example, a man charged with assaulting women showed "signs of mental disorder" in court. He was "very excitable" and exhibited erratic behavior. After a medical examination, two physicians declared him insane, noting that he was too "dangerous to be at large." In the course of the deliberations over his confinement, the colonial surgeon made a revealing comment about the purpose of the mental institution. He observed that "lunatics are put into an asylum not so much with regard to their own good and their ultimate cure, which is no doubt one object, as for the public protection and safety."[32] A

threat to life and property obviously aroused anxiety and necessitated prompt and strict measures to check the threat.

Prisoners in the Freetown Gaol suffering from mental disorders
were also sent to the asylum. An unusual case involved a man
serving a ten-year sentence for wounding a person with intent to
murder. He ran about naked in his cell, refused to speak, drank
his urine, tried to hide, and made distorted facial expressions.
This bizarre behavior caught the attention of the jail keeper, who
sent him to Kissy for observation. After seven days, the asylum
medical officer reported that the prisoner ate and slept well,
responded correctly to questions, displayed moderate nonviolent
behavior, and kept clean habits. He was certified sane and
returned to jail. Soon after, he refused to work or abide by prison
rules. At that point, he was sentenced to twelve lashes, the painful denouement of this case.[33]

In another instance, a prisoner serving six months for attempted arson had "a sudden attack of dementia," and was sent to
Kissy and certified insane. A few months later, his relatives petitioned the authorities, arguing that the man had recovered and
should be allowed to return home. Medical officials concurred,
noting he "is now fit to be discharged in care of his brother." In
fact, however, on the eve of his release, he had a violent fit, an
incident that cancelled all arrangements for his discharge.[34]

Some prisoners were shunted back and forth between jail and
asylum. A jail inmate engaged in violent or deviant behavior
would be removed to the asylum and placed under observation
and care. Over time, the person's conduct would moderate and
the prisoner would be returned to the jail, and the whole process
of removal and return would be repeated at some later date.[35] On
the other hand, many prisoners did recover from bouts with mental disturbance. When the terms of confinement expired, they
were formally certified sane and were discharged from the
asylum as well as from the jail.[36]

In the closing years of the nineteenth century, Kissy Lunatic
Asylum still received mentally ill people from all over British
West Africa, notably from the Gambia, the Gold Coast, and
Lagos. Colonial authorities often made arrangements by way of
the telegraph, with a simple terse request about accommodations.
For example, a telegram from the Gambia to the governor of
Sierra Leone asked: "Is there room for a hopeless lunatic at Kissy
Asylum?" The reply from Sierra Leone read: "There is room for
a hopeless lunatic at Kissy Asylum."[37]

Transported by ship, each insane patient was accompanied to
Freetown by two constables. While the voyage was usually un-

eventful, on occasion complications developed. One individual, arriving from the Gambia, was so weak and exhausted that he was carried on a stretcher to the Colonial Hospital in Freetown where, a few hours after admission, he died.[38]

An unfortunate accident led to the death of a "Lagos lunatic." This man displayed suicidal tendencies and was put in irons by the escorts and shackled to a winch. En route, steam was turned on to raise the anchor, and through the same pipe, steam was conveyed to the winch. The man had inadvertently opened the valve of the hoist with his feet. The winch went into motion, catching the man's arm between the wire and the drum, resulting in serious lacerations and a compound fracture of the right forearm. While the arm was bandaged in splints, it was several days before the ship arrived in Freetown. By that time, the arm became gangrenous and had to be amputated. The man died from the shock of the operation.[39]

This was an atypical case. Most of the mentally ill coming from other British colonies arrived safely, albeit few returned home: most of them died in the Kissy institution.[40] The majority of these patients suffered from severe disorders and were designated as suicidal or dangerous to others, or were identified as "criminally insane."[41] In 1887, seventy patients resided at the asylum, forty male and thirty female; of this group, seven came from the Gold Coast, two from Lagos, and one from the Gambia.[42] The number of foreign patients remained constant, varying between 10 and 15 percent of the total until the early 1900s, when asylums were well established in Lagos and the Gold Coast.

While the number of foreign inmates declined, the patient population of the asylum increased slowly: from 70 in 1887 to 119 in 1898 to 138 in 1917.[43] Around this time, the opening years of the twentieth century, the asylum received few patients from the protectorate, the interior of the country. Freetown and its environs supplied the bulk of the institution's clientele. Some of the characteristics of the patient population may be surmised from a 1902 medical report sent to England.

This document was a response to an inquiry from the London County Asylum, requesting information about insanity in Sierra Leone. It was based on a study of 105 patients at the Kissy asylum. The proportion of males to females was two to one, with seventy-seven males and thirty-eight females. In terms of ethnic identity, the largest number of mentally disturbed in this sample were Muslim Krios, or Aku. The Mende and the Temne, the two

largest ethnic groups in Sierra Leone, also had substantial numbers. And a few cases represented such smaller ethnic units as the
Susu, Kroo, Limba, and Loko.

The report offered an explanation for the large numbers of Aku
insane. Muslim Krios had achieved a higher level of education
and training than most other groups. Consequently, they experienced more stress and competition in "every walk of life." They
felt "domestic worry," "overwork," "mental anxiety." In contrast, other ethnic peoples, this study contended, including the
Mende and Temne, had few wants, engaged in menial tasks, and
encountered only minor mental strains. For this sector of society,
"intemperance in drink" was a chief cause of mental disorder.

Propinquity to the mental institution was another factor explaining the ethnic distribution of the sample. Most Aku lived in
Freetown, and some Temne and Mende came from the protectorate to the city, searching for any kind of work. Often they
remained unemployed and frustrated, and the police found them
"wandering about the streets." The report concluded that most of
these patients succumbed to the more violent forms of insanity,
namely acute and chronic mania.[44]

The classification of mental disorders in such general terms
was a characteristic of late-nineteenth century psychiatric nosol-
ogy. Patients at Kissy were assigned to psychiatric categories,
and, over the years, these nosological identifications confirmed
the findings of the 1902 medical report. The majority of patients
suffered from chronic mania. A significant number were associated with acute mania and subacute mania, and only a few were
labeled idiotic, or melancholic, or epileptic. Clearly, a large
number of violent patients were incarcerated at Kissy Lunatic
Asylum.[45]

Institutional deaths were attributed frequently to a psychiatric
disorder. An asylum report of 1892 listed twelve deaths occurring
during the year; seven from chronic mania, one from subacute
mania, three from acute mania, and one from dementia.[46] After
1900, with increased efficiency and sophistication in the medical
department, disease designations superceded general psychiatric
labels, and usually a specific illness was found to be the cause of
an inmate's death. Each death necessitated a coroner's inquest
and only a few were attributed to a psychiatric problem. "General
paralysis of the insane," a precisely understood brain disease,
later found to be tertiary syphilis, was the most obvious example.

Some of the more common causes of inmate fatality included
Bright's disease, nephritis, pulmonary tuberculosis, enteritis,

dysentery, apoplexy, anemia, and a condition called "exhaustion" or "general debility." There were also cases of trypanosomiasis.[47] The number of deaths occurring annually ranged from 15 to 20 percent of the total inmate population. In 1906, this trend was altered when over a third of the patients died, chiefly because of an epidemic of beriberi and dysentery.[48]

SOME IMPROVEMENTS - BUT LINGERING STAFF PROBLEMS

Some of the sicknesses and deaths at the asylum were attributed to the unsanitary, run-down condition of the buildings. The facility was termed "a disgrace to any civilized country," its continued existence excused only by the poor financial condition of the colony. Improvements seemed assured when, in 1898, the foundations of a new asylum were laid.[49] Progress remained slow, however, and it was not until 1910 that a new complex of buildings was completed. Some of the structures included cell blocks, a wash house, a latrine, kitchens, and a rebuilt administrative center. At the time, the resident medical officer commented that Sierra Leone now had "an asylum built in accordance with modern ideas and one which cannot fail to have a favorable effect on the health and general well-being of the patients."[50]

Around the turn of the century, the staff of the institution increased. In 1891, it consisted of a head keeper, two assistant keepers, two female nurses, two laborers, a cook, and six attendants. By 1910, a medical officer - an African physician trained in Great Britain - resided at Kissy. As the chief administrator, he supervised a staff enlarged to ten attendants, twelve laborers, a medical dispenser, two dressers, five female nurses, three cooks, and a laundress, as well as a keeper and an assistant keeper.[51]

The maintenance of staff order and discipline remained a problem. At times, an administrative policy of drift, or perhaps indifference, prevailed, and the staff received little direction or support. This fact, and the informal, loosely organized nature of institutional life, combined with the actions of incompetent staff members, fostered negligent and inferior care. Visiting medical officers complained about the difficulties of handling attendants who repeatedly ignored instructions. One physician noted that a number of practices could not be stopped: disregarding all his pleas and threats, some attendants persistently threw refuse in drains, allowed patients to drink dirty water, delayed posting books, and permitted stray dogs and fowls to loiter in the asylum yards.[52]

If threats or fines did not reform a recalcitrant staff member, continued or gross violations of rules of conduct caused an employee's dismissal. For example, over the years, an attendant committed a number of offenses, such as insubordination, carelessness on duty, misconduct, and ill-treatment of patients, including "striking a lunatic." Fined for each infraction, he paid a higher sum for any incident involving the mishandling of a patient. In the end, he was caught drunk on duty and was immediately dismissed.[53]

In another case, an assistant keeper of the asylum was removed from office for gross carelessness and neglect of duty. He disregarded an assignment to watch over some patients and went home, leaving the inmates without supervision. One of them escaped.[54] A criminal action brought another employee's dismissal. This worker sold the vegetables from the institution's garden and kept the money when the proceeds from the sale were supposed to go to the patients, allowing them to purchase luxury items. The man was taken into custody, charged with obtaining money under false pretenses, and eventually sentenced to four days in prison with hard labor.[55]

Acts of cruelty against inmates aroused particular concern. An unfortunate case involved an old, physically weak patient who did not want a bath. Offended by this refusal, the attendant and two assistants dragged the inmate on "stoney ground" to a cell, where he was kicked and beaten. The day after the incident, the man could not walk, his feet remained swollen, his back was badly bruised, and he had severe body pains. The medical officer called the matter "a very brutal act to a poor insane and convalescent man" and warned that such cruelty could have killed the patient. The guilty attendant was fired, and the two assistants were fined three days pay and severely reprimanded.[56]

Medical authorities in Freetown expressed considerable indignation over a case dealing with an unexpected pregnancy of an asylum patient. The apparent culprit, an attendant in the male wards, escaped punishment. He left the institution and faded into society when the incident became public knowledge. The visiting medical officer took harsh criticism for failing to detect the pregnancy, even when it had advanced beyond six months. The final resolutions on this matter curtly stated that "his application for increased pay will not be entertained" and "any further dereliction

on duty will render his retention in the service undesirable."
Other responsible asylum officials were penalized: the keeper, the
matron, and her assistants were reprimanded and fined, in incre-
ments to be deducted over several months. This whole affair also
marked the beginning of the end for the keeper. Authorities knew
about his negligence and lax security; he allowed unauthorized
persons access to the keys of the institution, including the
women's areas. His refusal to change this policy led to his dismissal.[57]

Occasionally incidents occurred that demonstrated a bad practice or faulty policy but could not be charged to any one person's
negligence or incompetence. An unusual and dramatic example
took place soon after an unstable, violent patient picked out a
piece of iron from a pile of rubbish in the asylum yard. This person fashioned the iron object into a crude knife. During a fight
with an inmate, he stabbed his opponent. At the time of the incident, a medical officer was in a building nearby and was called to
the scene. He observed two men lying on the ground; the attacker
apparently suffering from a blow to the head, the other man had
a "wound on the right side of the body from which a coil of large
intestine about a foot in length was protruding."

Assuming this man would die unless he quickly received
surgery, the physician telegraphed higher authorities in Freetown
and gained permission to operate. He cleaned the sand and dirt
off the intestine, enlarged the opening, placed the gut back into
the abdomen, and closed the wound with silk sutures. In his
report, the physician referred to the rubbish heaps around the
asylum grounds, noting that they offered "opportunity to evilly
disposed lunatics to injure either themselves or others." This affair dramatized a bad practice that officials had overlooked during this time of institutional renovations. Thereafter, building
materials and trash were kept beyond the reach of patients.[58]

In the mid- and late 1920s, admissions to the asylum gradually
increased: the number of patients housed and treated annually
rose from 144 in 1924 to 160 in 1928 to 175 in 1930.[59] Patients
still came from the Gambia, but were no longer sent from Lagos
or the Gold Coast. The hospital administration now resisted pressure to admit mentally ill persons from the protectorate, observing that the institution was not large enough for all the insane in
the country. Any mentally ill native of Freetown and environs,
even if living in the protectorate, was eligible for admission to
Kissy. The asylum door, however, was not shut completely to
persons from the hinterland; at his discretion, the chief medical

officer had the authority to admit some patients from the protectorate.[60]

TOWARD A MENTAL HOSPITAL

In late 1928, a major pressure for change and reform came
from England. This was a directive pamphlet entitled "Some Suggestions Regarding the Administration of Colonial Mental Hospitals," written by J. R. Lord, a former president of the Royal
Medico-Psychological Association and secretary of the National
Council for Mental Hygiene. It outlined guidelines and recom-
mendations for mental hospitals located throughout the British
Empire. The authorities in Freetown, however, made only a
guarded response to it.[61]

First and foremost, Lord stressed that the treatment of mental
disorder remained the basic objective of a mental institution.
Moreover, a hospital was an independent facility, divorced from
police or correctional agencies. Operating according to modern
hospital and nursing ideals and practices, he continued, the institution should use the most simplified procedures for admissions
and discharges and encourage voluntary admission. It should
keep a chiefly nonresident staff, a proven policy that militates
against the formation of rigid institutional routines and behavior.
In line with psychiatric practice in other areas of the world,
notably England and the United States, such terms as asylum and
lunatic were obsolete. An asylum was now called a mental hospital, a lunatic was a mentally ill person. The new terms were, of
course, designed to remove some of the stigma associated with
caring for the mentally disordered.[62]

While demanding these nomenclature changes, Lord specified
the need for more female nurses and for a medical officer with
psychiatric experience. He stressed the importance of appointing
responsible citizens to a "visiting committee" that would inspect
the institution periodically and report to the colonial governor. In
effect, the committee would allay public suspicions and prejudice
against the hospital. Along with this committee, the appointment
of voluntary "lady visitors" to the hospital would promote good
relations between the institution and the community, as well as
improve patient morale.

Lord was sensitive to the overcrowded conditions in colonial
institutions, and he offered remedies: chronic, harmless patients
could be paroled or boarded out with suitable families; quiet,

nonoffensive, physically sick or infirm patients could be quartered temporarily or permanently at the colonial hospital. At the same time, the mental hospital, he said, must maintain a policy accommodating only those patients requiring active care and treatment. A basic classification policy of segregating acute and chronic patients must be observed. The noisy and turbulent patients should be removed to special areas and returned to a quiet setting only when their excitement had abated and self-control returned. Lord also recommended more lay authority over the detention and discharge of inmates, particularly with "un-recovered" patients.[63]

The colonial administration in Freetown accepted readily the name change, dropping "asylum" for "mental hospital." Some of Lord's other proposals, however, presented difficulties. The call for more female nurses was viewed as not applicable to Sierra Leone because "there are no African female nurses with anything like the qualifications necessary." The recommendation that harmless, long-term patients be placed with receptive families was also received cooly. Experience demonstrated that only friends and relatives of a patient gave proper supervision and care. And the notion that laypersons exercise more authority over the custody and release of patients was dismissed: existing legis-lation controlled the procedures, and there was no sentiment for change in Sierra Leone.[64]

The implementation of Lord's suggestions for the appointment of lady visitors and a visiting committee received unexpected community support, surprising the authorities. Volunteers willing to serve the mental hospital seemed a most unlikely prospect; one administrator did not believe "such people could be found in Sierra Leone."[65]

This was soon proved an unfounded assumption. The govern-ment sent inquiries to several associations in Freetown and Kissy, including the Bathurst Street Association, the Michael Cottage Society, the W. C. Associates, the Truscott Society, and the Holy Trinity Dorcas; the response disclosed that many of these com-munity groups already maintained ties with the mental hospital. Each one supplied either the name of an individual or a list of persons who would be delighted to serve as a visitor.

The members of one association, known as the Charity Board, kept written accounts of their visits and submitted reports to the director of medical services in Freetown. They interacted only with female patients, mingling and conversing with them, and taking messages to their relatives. Some of the inmates were "wild, rough, and uncontrollable" and disrupted gatherings; still, the Charity Board held that the visits were beneficial to the women, by keeping them in contact with their families. Its success with entertaining the women led the organization to request permission to visit with male patients. Authorities accepted this demand, but restricted visits to mild-mannered men, and allowed them to be seen only in the waiting room.

The Charity Board also responded to the complaints of patients. For example, some inmates protested about the policy of serving only two meals a day, claiming that they suffered hunger pangs because the interval between meals was too long. This complaint was relayed to the administration, and apparently action was taken. After their next visit, Board members recorded that the well-being of the patients showed a "remarkable improvement."

On New Year's Day, 1930, the Charity Board staged a major social event at Kissy, entertaining and distributing provisions to over 200 patients. Such an event, coupled with the positive interactions between mental patients and the members of other associations, elicited praise from the administration. One colonial secretary commented that the experience with lady visitors "has proved successful to a greater extent than I anticipated." [66]

In addition to the Charity Board, a visiting committee was organized at Kissy in 1928. It held regular meetings, averaging four or five a year, and influenced institutional programs and policy until the late 1930s. Its membership varied between six and eight persons: a police magistrate, a clergyman, two or four laypersons, and two physicians. For a few years, one of the hospital's medical officers, M.C.F. Easmon, a Sierra Leonean doctor and specialist in psychiatric disorders, played a key role in the committee's deliberations.

At every committee meeting, the members toured the facility, commenting on conditions. They inspected the kitchen and paid special attention to the preparation of food for the patients. They noticed the effect of any change in the physical plant: a new partition in the male compound, for example, facilitated the segregation of the violent, noisy inmates from the quiet ones. The committee reported that the partition brought a "decided improvement in the condition of the patients," and recommended that a similar wall be constructed in the female compound. The committee also recognized that the visits of members of community support groups had a positive influence on inmates. It expressed delight over the increasing number of callers: warm endorsements and appreciation went to the lady visitors and members of religious associations who devoted their time to entertaining the patients.[67]

The physical health of the inmates remained the committee's basic concern. Its reports indicated usually that the hospital was "clean and in good order"; the health of patients was "good" or "generally satisfactory." There were times, however, when health matters aroused "grave concern." A large number of deaths in 1931, for example, prompted an inquiry. The investigation revealed that several deaths resulted from pericarditis; others were attributed to "some disease brought about by faulty feeding," a revelation that caused demands for a flexible, more varied diet and fresher supplies of rice.[68]

In 1932, several fatalities led to another investigation. M.C.F. Easmon, the leading medical officer at the hospital, reported that only a few of these deaths warranted special comment: these were fatal cases of gastroenteritis. The postmortem examination of one person revealed "an unusually heavy infection of round worms"; another case was complicated by pneumonia; others were short-term patients admitted in poor condition who had such "filthy habits" as "eating the dressings applied to their wounds and licking up the discharges."[69] Two years later, in 1934, the institutional death rate was again slightly higher than normal and this fact drew attention. Since most of the fatalities were failing elderly men, no investigation occurred.[70]

Administrators remained attentive to the etiology of inmate mortality. With greater medical specificity than in the past, annual reports identified the cause of a patient's death without reference to any psychiatric disorder. Some of the causes included pulmonary tuberculosis, bronchopneumonia, lobar pneumonia, gastroenteritis, subacute nephritis, amoebic dysentery, and myocardial degeneration.[71] Unexpected events interrupted the calm of administrative routine. A violent death, for example, led to an inquest: a female inmate was killed when another patient smashed a large stone into her head. The investigative report expressed regret over this incident, and a jury recommended that the hospital yards be kept clean of stones that could be used as weapons.[72]

An investigation also followed any incidence of widespread sickness. Over the years, a continuing problem at the mental hospital was outbreaks of beriberi; an institutional epidemic occurred in early 1940. The root cause of the trouble was bad rice, which was "old, broken, full of weevils, and unfit for use in a closed institution." The rice had been milled three times, losing its nutritional value. In addition, the supply of greens to the hospital was inadequate, providing no supplement to the daily fare. Such a badly balanced diet, the investigators concluded, accounted for the outbreak of sickness. Eight patients had symptoms of paraplegic beriberi - inability or difficulty in standing or walking, no knee jerks, and tenderness of the calf muscle. One died; the others received injections of vitamin B1 and showed marked improvement. The medical officer began daily examinations of all patients, and the institutional diet was monitored carefully. As a result of these measures, the seven patients recovered completely from the disease and no new cases of beriberi occurred.[73]

Under Easmon's direction, the visiting committee encouraged a policy of keeping patients occupied with constructive work, particularly if the labor brought a profit to the institution. Gardening was a successful enterprise. Basket making, another occupational activity, required instruction and took time to develop. Medical authorities argued that basket work had special therapeutic value, noting that it aroused and kept the patients' interest. For a few years, the baskets made at Kissy were sold to the sanitation department. Woodcutting proved the most profitable patient activity. A committee report observed that it had reached "gratifying dimensions," and it remained productive, with several cords of wood supplied regularly to other medical facilities in Kissy and Freetown.[74]

Another important part of the committee's work involved acting on patient requests and complaints. The most frequent demands of inmates concerned maintaining contacts with relatives. Easmon responded by making inquiries about the location of families and the willingness of relatives to visit the mental hospital. In some instances, he achieved success and established a pattern of family calls. On other occasions, he found that relatives no longer accepted responsibility for the patient. This was usually the case with a long-term inmate who had lost ties with friends and family.[75]

RETRENCHMENT

A related and equally difficult situation concerned the discharge of recovered patients who had no home. While these inmates had gained sufficient mental health to be released, they had no place to go. An old soldier from Jamaica, for example, had no friends or relatives in Sierra Leone; a man from the interior was not wanted in his village; the relatives of another man would not take him back. The first two of these cases were resolved: the government of Jamaica accepted the soldier, and the chief of the up-country village took charge of the patient, a former townsman. The third man remained in the hospital, which elicited warnings about the harm wrought by keeping patients institutionalized. Such persons became discontented and could not achieve a complete restoration of mental health.[76]

The pressure to find places for recovered homeless inmates reflected a new policy of retrenchment that began in the 1930s. This policy also curtailed plans for enlarging the institution. In the spring of 1929, a project to expand the hospital was outlined in a detailed government report, originating in the office of the Director of Public Works and sent to the Director of Medical Services, which specified the options for constructing an extension of the mental hospital. While much of this document focused on determining the best place to build an addition, a few assumptions were made: the asylum appeared congested, particularly the male wards; an extension was "urgently required;" further construction would be needed within five years; and it was presumed that, if the present rate of increase of patients continued, six additional wards would be built over a period of fifteen years.

This proposal received little response, and met repeated delays. In 1930, the government postponed the plan, noting that a "need for economy" would hold off action in 1930 and 1931. In July 1932, the matter ended with the declaration: "There is no present need to consider an extension." The hospital was no longer overcrowded. An unusually high annual death rate, coupled with an aggressive discharge policy, had reduced sharply the number of patients.[77]

In line with its forceful release program, the hospital administration was successful in a trial or probation discharge policy involving patients with cooperating families. Administrators also monitored closely the admittance and release of non-Sierra Leonean inmates. A report on patients from the Gambia in the Kissy hospital, for example, was sent to the colonial secretary in December 1930. It identified nine Gambians, six male and three female, and analyzed carefully the physical and mental condition of each inmate, noting the date of admission as well as the prognosis for discharge. Of the nine inmates, only one, a 36-year-old man, was deemed fit for release and repatriation to the Gambia. He talked "intelligently," was "well-behaved and obedient to asylum discipline," and had "recovered his mental balance." The other eight patients displayed erratic, often violent, behavior and had little awareness of their condition or surroundings.[78] Such odds, only one out of nine returning home, were typical, making the control of admissions more important than the release of cured patients.

The policy of retrenchment at the mental hospital, so evidenced by the rejection of plans for expansion, the strict regulation of the numbers of admissions, and the encouragement of early discharges, stemmed directly from the great economic depression of the 1930s. This was a time of financial stringency and instability in the global economy, and the economic difficulties in the United Kingdom adversely affected the economy of Sierra Leone. Outside support waned, and self-sufficiency, the basic colonial policy, could not be maintained. The country could not support itself, and colonial authorities demanded drastic reductions in expenditures.

A memorandum from the colonial secretary in Freetown, dated September 16, 1932, addressed the subject of "Public Expenditures on Government Medical Services in Sierra Leone." The secretary reported that the current funds allotted for such public health matters were "quite unjustified": Sierra Leone was a "poor colony," and its expenditures for social services were out of proportion to the country's resources. In 1931, revenue had fallen by 32 percent of the 1928 estimates; while some improvement came in 1932, income was down still by 15 percent of the 1928 figure, and further cutbacks were necessary.[79]

A new policy was needed, the colonial secretary argued, one that encouraged private medical practice to develop an alternative to continued and expensive government outlays for health services. There were precedents for this change: just as private contractors handled projects for the Public Works Department, so medical practitioners must take over services now performed solely by the government. Such a policy would help relieve the financial burden of the Medical Department, as well as enhance the status of private practitioners. During this time of economic troubles, the colonial secretary insisted, the government must support the country's professional class. It must provide opportunity for educated citizens: an unemployed class of doctors, or lawyers, or other trained persons, he warned, would pose "a serious danger to the state."

Accordingly, the secretary declared that the Medical Department would no longer provide all of the health services of the community. Its activities would be reduced, those of the private sector expanded and strengthened. For example, no vacancies in the Medical Department, aside from the senior medical officer, would be filled in the future; a retainer system, a method of giving contracts to individuals for specific services, would direct African medical officers toward the private sector; and young European doctors, at the onset of their careers, would be encouraged to come and engage in private practice in Sierra Leone. In the more remote areas of the country, a policy of providing subsidies to medical missions would provide adequate public health services to the population and eliminate the need for maintaining small government hospitals. All of these measures, the colonial secretary concluded, would not cut down medical benefits. Instead, extravagance would be reduced and there would be greater economy in the administration, allowing the government to focus on the essential tasks of maintaining the system in a time of economic stress.[80]

MODERNIZATION, OVERCROWDING, ECONOMIC MALAISE

During and after World War II, the economy of Sierra Leone improved. Iron ore and diamond mining in the interior stimulated growth; Freetown grew in size and population. The British government, authorized by the Colonial Development and Welfare Acts, initiated projects to better the condition of roads, schools, and medical and welfare agencies. Postwar prosperity brought change to the mental hospital. The facility was modernized and renovated: electricity was installed, and a loud speaker system was set up. Plans for extending the building were prepared again, and this time were approved by the authorities.

Some things did not change: the encouragement of occupational therapy remained a basic administrative endeavor. Gardening, basket-, mattress-, and pillow-making, tailoring, and domestic tasks such as laundering and assisting in the kitchen kept receptive patients occupied. The patient mortality rate remained constant, and the types of death fell into three groups: one associated with old age, consisting of cerebral hemorrhage and thrombosis cases; a second group with neurosyphilis; and the third group, embracing intestinal disorders, notably the dysenteries and helminthic infestations.

Overcrowding, a new development, became a major problem. The hospital was designed for around 100 patients. In 1948, it accommodated 176 inmates, 189 resided in 1949, and 191 in 1951. The congestion created a destructive institutional milieu that constricted the living and recreational areas of patients and frustrated the policy of segregating inmates by behavior. The violent, criminal, and offensive patients were frequently quartered with inmates who were merely under observation or were suffering from mild, treatable disorders. Such circumstances hampered treatment efforts and diminished the chances for recovery.[81]

The overcrowded conditions can be explained. The growth of the population of Freetown and environs brought a corresponding increase in the number of mentally ill persons. Also, beginning in the 1950s, significantly large numbers of patients were sent to Kissy from the interior of the country. Sensitive to this trend, the British, in the years before independence, suggested the possibility of building a mental hospital in the protectorate.[82]

During the 1960s, when Sierra Leone became an independent nation-state, the idea of establishing another asylum was dropped, and Kissy Mental Hospital became a national depository for mentally ill persons. The ability to serve the entire nation, in effect, the movement of patients to and from the institution and the provinces, was facilitated by improved communication and transportation networks. The steady flow of mentally ill persons, however, coming from the interior as well as the traditional catchment area of Freetown, kept the hospital crowded. In spite of the construction of additions to the facility, conditions worsened.

Other developments exacerbated the overcrowding and complicated the admissions and discharge process. Chronic, long-term cases accumulated; these patients had been abandoned and forgotten by their families. They took on the symptoms of institutionalization and became totally dependent on the hospital for maintenance and custody. An increasing number of readmissions created another problem for the administration. A revolving-door pattern of admissions and discharges, a basic trend occurring in many Western mental hospitals, was established at Kissy. Such patients were received, treated or constrained, and then sent home several times over a period of months and years. This situation stigmatized them as insane persons to the wider community and raised questions about the nature and effectiveness of treatment programs.

A more disturbing trend, over which the administration lacked firm controls, was the growing number of criminally insane entering and remaining in the hospital. Police and correctional authorities throughout the country sent criminals who displayed erratic, and particularly violent, behavior to Kissy for observation. This prevailing practice was abused frequently, burdening the institution with persons who had violated laws but were not mentally ill. Their presence demanded special security precautions and arrangements and diverted effort and attention away from the basic therapeutic role of the hospital.[83]

Throughout the 1970s, all of the problems concomitant with the congested facilities continued to plague the institution. Conditions deteriorated further with the decline of the country's economy. A change in the hospital administration, however, occurring in 1981, led to the inauguration of a new policy aimed at relieving the vexations of an overcrowded institution. The major feature of the change was a simplified admissions procedure. An individual was no longer required to be certified insane by a physician. Before 1981, each patient received a certificate of emergency, previously labeled a certificate of lunacy, which specified the evidence of the client's mental state. This was the formal means to admit a client to the hospital. Adherence to the procedure hardened; once admitted, many patients became long-term cases, difficult to discharge to any responsible relative or authority.

Under the new policy, in contrast, patients came directly to the institution for assessment, accompanied by a close relative or friend. A psychiatric examination was conducted, and, if the patient required institutionalization, a contract was concluded between the relative and the psychiatrist, the director of the mental hospital, specifying three months as the maximum time that the patient would remain in the hospital. This arrangement sought to discourage persons from dumping a mentally ill family member in the institution for a long-term stay.

Other measures designed to restrict admissions involved children under 12 years of age and elderly persons over 65. Such cases would not be hospitalized but treated at home or at an outpatient clinic. Also under the new policy, the criminally insane would be kept in a special psychiatric facility in prison rather than being sent to Kissy. These changes in admissions policy decreased the number of patients entering the hospital, easing the burdens of managing an overcrowded institution.[84]

Limiting admissions, however, could not overcome the most fundamental problem that thwarted effective institutional care - the depressed economy. On this matter, the experience of Sierra Leone followed a worldwide pattern. Governments across the globe viewed mental health care as a low priority item. Even in the best of times, in periods of economic boom, public funds allocated to mental institutions usually are insufficient to initiate major change or innovation. With economic downturns, the situation worsens, and policy focuses solely on maintaining the existing hospital system. Throughout colonial times as well as during the period since independence, the fortunes of Kissy Mental Hospital have related directly to the state of the country's economy. Toward the end of the twentieth century, the general economic malaise of the nation continued to impose stringencies on the government, restricting funding of the hospital, which severely curtailed programs and narrowed policy options.

NOTES

1. Christopher Fyfe, *A History of Sierra Leone* (London: Oxford University Press, 1962), 138-39.
2. Fyfe, *A History of Sierra Leone*, 134, 159-60, 172, 208-9, 229.
3. Ibid., 267; National Archives of Sierra Leone, Freetown (hereafter cited as SLA), Governor's Dispatches to Secretary of State, 1846-1847, Numbers 46, 94, 106.
4. George James Moutafakis, *The British Colonial Policy and Administration of the British West African Settlements, 1866-1888* (Ph.D. diss., New York University, 1960), 369-70; Philip D. Curtin, *The Image of Africa: British Ideas and Action, 1780-1850* (Madison: University of Wisconsin Press, 1964), 349-52. Ranklin was the author of *The White Man's Grave: A Visit to Sierra Leone in 1834* (London 1836), 2 vols.
5. Moutafakis, *British Colonial Policy and Administration*, 180-82.
6. Philip D. Curtin, "Medical Knowledge and Urban Planning in Tropical Africa," *American Historical Review* 90 (June 1985): 594-613; Leo Spitzer, "The Mosquito and Segregation in Sierra Leone," *Canadian Journal of African Studies* 2 (1968): 49-61; Leo Spitzer, *The Creoles of Sierra Leone: Responses to Colonialism, 1870-1945* (Madison: University of Wisconsin Press, 1974), 51-9. An excellent comparative study of the death rates of Europeans in tropical parts of the nineteenth century world is Philip D. Curtin, *Death by Migration* (New York: Cambridge University Press, 1989).
7. Spitzer, *The Creoles of Sierra Leone*, 59.
8. Moutafakis, *British Colonial Policy and Administration*,

50-51, 59, 120-21, 339.

9. Curtin, *The Image of Africa*, 195-96.

10. D. C. Howard and A. I. Payne, "Deforestation, the Decline of the Horse, and the Spread of the Tsetse Fly and Trypanosomiasis (Nagana) in Nineteenth Century Sierra Leone," *Journal of African History* 16 (1975): 239-56.

11. SLA, CSO 1059/1884 Rules for the Guidance and Governance of the Medical Department of Sierra Leone, June 1882.

12. SLA, CSO 1059/1884; SLA, CSO 2607/1887 Report on the Various Hospitals in Freetown and Kissy, 3 September 1887.

13. SLA, CSO 1959/1884.

14. Ibid.; SLA, CSO 1584/1883, 3 July 1883; CSO 3416/1893 Annual Report of the Medical Department of Sierra Leone for 1892.

15. SLA, CSO 1358/1882 Letter, 20 July 1882.

16. SLA, CSO 3321/1883 Letter, 23 March 1883.

17. SLA, CSO 3416/1893 Annual Report.

18. Examples of matters related to repairs and maintenance of the facility include: SLA, CSO 1476/1882; 996/1883; 1125/1884; 1295/1884; 456/1885; 6015/1889; 3894/1889; 2820/1893; 2953/1893; 56/1894; 1477/1894; 2058/1894.

19. SLA, CSO 3365/1887 Escape of Two Lunatics from the Kissy Asylum, 25 November 1887.

20. SLA, CSO 444/1883 Escape of a Female Lunatic from the Asylum, 26 March 1883.

21. SLA, CSO 1115/1900 Escape of Lunatic, 3 April 1900.

22. SLA, CSO 1783/1901 Escape of Lunatic, 18 April 1901.

23. SLA, CSO 3972/1900 Escape of a Lunatic from the Lunatic Asylum at Kissy, 27 December 1900; CSO 1912 MP M1-100 Number 16/12 Escape of a Male Lunatic from the Kissy Asylum, 3 January 1912; CSO 1914 MP Number 190/1914 Escape of a Female Lunatic from the Asylum on 20 January, 21 January 1914.

24. SLA, CSO 2050/1904 Escape of a Female Lunatic from the Female to the Male Division of Asylum, 16 May 1904; 1856/1906 Escape of a Lunatic from the Asylum at Kissy, 24 April 1906; 1661/1907 Escape of Lunatic, 25 April 1907; 213/1880 Letter, 15 March 1880.

25. SLA, CSO 138/1879 Lunatic Release from Asylum Recommended, 17 March 1874; CSO 140/1879 Joseph B. Cole, Lunatic, 10 March 1879, 13 March 1879.

26. SLA, CSO 939/1884 Petition from Son to Place Mother in the Asylum, 30 July 1884.

27. SLA, CSO 277/1878 W.A.H. Smith Asking for Confinement of His Brother at the Lunatic Asylum at Kissy, 30 May

1878.

28. SLA, CSO 82/1881 J. A. Dayrell Wants Removal of His Son from Lunatic Asylum Kissy, 18 February 1881.

29. SLA, CSO 313/1878 Daniel Johnson, Patient, Lunatic Asylum Elizabeth Taylor, His Sister Asks for His Removal, 11 July 1878, 13 July 1878.

30. SLA, CSO 3405/1900 Removal of Harriett Carr from Lunatic Asylum Solicited, 17 November 1900.

31. SLA, CSO Removal of Lunatic, 5 September 1885.

32. SLA, CSO Rhodes - a Lunatic, 21 August 1887, 21 October 1887.

33. SLA, CSO 1913 MP M181-248 Number 2286 Authority for the Removal of the Prisoner Beareh to the Lunatic Asylum, 21 October 1913.

34. SLA, CSO M24/17 Insane Condition of Sandi, 31 January 1917.

35. SLA, CSO 2799/1887 Prisoner D. George Apparently Insane, 28 September 1887.

36. SLA, CSO 1917 M/PM 101-M/PM 182 Number PMO 359/17, 20 July 1917.

37. SLA, CSO 4913/1902 Accommodation for Gambia Lunatic, 4 December 1902.

38. SLA, CSO 625/1892 8 February 1892.

39. SLA, CSO 4010/1906 Accommodation for Two Male Lunatics from Lagos, 25 August 1906.

40. Examples of death notices: SLA, CSO 4552/1900; 3639/1905; 995/1905; 1983/1905; 2039/1906; 3265/1906; 3703/1906; 3728/1906; 3933/1906; 5316/1906; 3511/1907; 388/1909; 1681/1909.

41. SLA, CSO 869/1883 Return of Male Lunatics Transferred from Lagos Gaol to Sierra Leone, 19 July 1883; 1617/1885 Arrival of Lunatics. Three from Gold Coast. Two from Lagos, 12 July 1885; 710/1885 Lunatics from Lagos, 28 October 1885; 426/1886 Lunatic from Gambia, 2 March 1886; 1574/1892 Reception of Lunatic Prisoner into Kissy Asylum, 9 April 1892; 3787/1900 Admittance of a Lunatic Prisoner from Lagos into the Asylum at Kissy, 12 December 1900; 1268/1905 A Lunatic Sent for Confinement in Lunatic Asylum, Kissy by the Gambia Government, 16 March 1905; 5060/1906 Accommodation for a Female Lunatic Prisoner, 9 October 1906.

42. SLA, CSO 2607/1887 Report on the Various Hospitals in Freetown and Kissy, 3 September 1887.

43. Ibid.; SLA, CSO 1370/1900 Annual Medical Report 1898, 26 April 1900; SLA, CSO MP Number 49/1918 Medical and Sanitary Report 1917.

44. SLA, CSO 4405/1902 Particulars on Insanity Among Natives in Answer to Questions from London County Asylum, England, 15 October 1902.

45. SLA, CSO 1248/1902 Annual Medical Report 1900; 1352/1902 Annual Report of the Medical Department 1901.

46. SLA, CSO 3416/1893 Annual Report of the Medical Department 1892.

47. SLA, CSO 1919/1907 Annual Report of the Medical Department 1906; 2387/1908 Annual Report of the Medical Department 1907; Annual Medical and Sanitary Report for 1909; 1912 MP M101-M180 M111 Annual Medical and Sanitary Report for 1911; 1915 MP M1-M100 M98 Annual Medical Report for the Year Ending 31 December 1914; 1918 MP M205 Number 49/1918 Annual Medical and Sanitary Report 1917.

48. Annual Report of the Medical and Sanitary Department 1906.

49. SLA, CSO 1370/1900 Annual Medical Report, 26 April 1900.

50. SLA, CSO Annual Report of the Medical Department for the Year Ended 31 December 1910.

51. SLA, CSO 543/1892 Board on Hospitals and Lunatic Asylum, 2 February 1892; Annual Report of the Medical Department for the Year Ended 31 December 1910.

52. SLA, CSO 5390/1903 Petition of Staff of Female Lunatic Asylum Against Punishment Inflicted on Them by Dr. Gray, MO, 21 December 1903.

53. SLA, CSO 4011/1906 Dismissal of Attendant, 31 August 1906.

54. SLA, CSO 1857/1893 11 April 1893.

55. SLA, CSO 937/1906 Irregular Disposing of Vegetables by Attendant, 21 February 1906.

56. SLA, CSO 1912 M39 Number 313/1912 Charge of Cruelty Against Attendants, 7 February 1912.

57. SLA, CSO 3731/1902 Lunatic Patient, Susannah Morrison, Kissy Asylum, State of Pregnancy, 6 September 1902.

58. SLA, CSO 435/1904 Serious Affray Between Two Lunatics in Asylum, Kissy, 28 January 1904. The matter ended on a happy note: the victim of the stabbing survived, and two months after the incident, the physician reported that the patient's wound had healed and he was doing well.

59. Annual Medical and Sanitary Report 1924; SLA, CSO M126/29 Annual Medical and Sanitary Report for 1928, Annual Report of the Medical and Sanitary Department 1930.

60. SLA, CSO 2804/1921 Admission of Natives to the Kissy Lunatic Asylum, 2 September 1921.

61. SLA, CSO M12/29 Some Suggestions Regarding the Administration of Colonial Mental Hospitals by Lt. Col. J. R. Lord, 27 September 1928.

62. Ibid.

63. Ibid.

64. Ibid.

65. Ibid.; Correspondence 18 February 1929, 19 February 1929.

66. SLA, CSO M12/29; Correspondence 16 May 1929, 31 May 1929, 21 October 1929, 14 February 1930, 17 February 1930.

67. SLA, CSO M52/29 Report of Kissy Asylum Visiting Committee.

68. SLA, CSO M52/29 Minutes 23 December 1931.

69. SLA, CSO M52/29 Report on Fatal Cases of Gastroenteritis for Quarter ending September 21, 1931.

70. SLA, CSO M52/29 Minutes 4 October 1934.

71. SLA, CSO M49/31 Annual Medical and Sanitary Report 1931; Annual Report of the Medical and Sanitary Department for the Year 1932; Annual Report of the Medical and Sanitary Department for the Year 1935; Annual Report of the Medical and Sanitary Department for the Year 1936; Annual Report of the Medical Services 1937.

72. SLA, CSO M25/34 Lunatic Asylum Safeguards Against Injuries to Inmates, 28 June 1940.

73. SLA, CSO M13/40 Beri-Beri in the Kissy Lunatic Asylum, 8 February 1940, 28 June 1940.

74. SLA, CSO M52/29 Report of Kissy Asylum Visiting Committee, Minutes 9 July 1932, 27 September 1932, 21 December 1932, 25 June 1934, 4 October 1934, 10 January 1935, 26 June 1935, 25 September 1935, 23 December 1935.

75. SLA, CSO M52/29 Minutes 2 November 1929, 7 January 1931, 14 July 1931.

76. SLA, CSO M52/29 Minutes 29 December 1933, 28 March 1934.

77. SLA, CSO M39/32 Proposed Extension of Kissy Asylum, 15 April 1929.

78. SLA, CSO M43/29 Admissions and Discharges of Lunatics from the Gambia, 8 December 1930.

79. SLA, CSO M137/32 Public Expenditures on Government Medical Services in Sierra Leone, 16 September 1932.

80. SLA, CSO 177/32 Government Medical Services New Policy, 14 December 1932.

81. *Annual Report on Sierra Leone for the Year 1948* (London: His Majesty's Stationery Office), 31; *Annual Report on*

Sierra Leone for the Year 1954, 57-61; *Annual Report on Sierra Leone for the Year 1956*, 63-69; *Annual Report on Sierra Leone for the Year 1957*, 66-78; *Annual Report on the Medical and Health Services for the Year 1949 (Freetown)*; relevant also are the reports from the years 1949, 1952, 1953, 1954, 1957.

82. *Annual Report of the Medical and Health Services for the Year 1954*.

83. Author's analysis of cases of the 1960s, records in Kissy Mental Hospital.

84. E. H. Nahim, "Management of Patients from 1981"; written report of the director of Kissy Mental Hospital to the author, 1986.

4 The Patients

During the colonial era of twentieth century Sierra Leone, the patients at the Kissy asylum were given psychiatric designations in line with the general patterns established in British and other Western mental health facilities. An exception to this policy rested with a few patients identified with the tropical disease trypanosomiasis. Over time, the psychiatric categories changed; the prevailing terminology related to the emerging sophistication of psychiatry as well as the experience of the medical personnel at the Kissy hospital. The psychiatric designations applied to the patients ranged across the manias and the dementias, and included such categories as epilepsy, mental retardation, alcoholism, and drug addiction. After about 1940, delusional insanity and schizophrenia were used with increasing frequency. The largest number of patients, however, received no psychiatric designation at all.[1]

The inmates at Kissy reflected the ethnic and class mixture of the wider society, notably of Freetown and the western part of the country. This region was close to the asylum and, as noted, it served as a natural catchment area for the institution. Many Krios resided in Freetown and environs, a fact accounting for their significant numbers sent to the hospital. The two largest ethnic groups, the Mende and the Temne, had the greatest number of clients; those peoples far removed from Freetown, namely the Kissi and the Koranko, had the smallest representation of patients. But regardless of ethnic ties, the patients shared a dominant characteristic - low economic and social status. The institution housed predominantly the poor and the poverty-stricken, a large sector of the society of colonial Sierra Leone.

The case records of Kissy asylum patients constitute a substantial body of information from which the basic characteristics of the institution's clientele can be ascertained. In these documents, a client was often identified with a psychiatric designation; other fundamental data dealt with the individual's gender, age, religion, occupation, ethnic group, and length of institutionalization. Often, an inmate's profile was amplified further with a description of the patient's general demeanor. This information, synthesized and broken down into diagnostic areas, presents a unique portrait of mental and social disorder in colonial Sierra Leone.

TRYPANOSOMIASIS

Trypanosomiasis remained a threat to human life in early-twentieth-century Sierra Leone. Between 1905 and 1959, ten patients, eight men and two women, with this affliction were present at the asylum. The disease, notably after it caused permanent cerebral damage, produced clinical symptoms of schizophrenia, especially of the paranoid type.[2] Each case at Kissy followed a general pattern of behavior and was accompanied by the individual's physical deterioration. Usually such persons were incarcerated for reasons typical of most patients entering the institution. The individual was reported to be "troublesome," "violent," "fighting in the streets," "throwing stones at passersby," or "disturbing the public." A few of them were noisy and unruly at another hospital or infirmary and were transferred to the asylum.

After admission, this type of difficult behavior initially bothered others, but within a few weeks, the patient's conduct underwent a dramatic change. Listlessness, lack of energy, and loss of vitality became the most obvious manifestations of the transformation. The inmate slept most of the time and had "to be roused to take food." There were attempts to arrest the degenerative course of the disease, largely to stimulate the central nervous system by means of hypodermic injections of strychnine. Invariably, the condition worsened; the individual sunk into a semicomatose condition, developed bed sores, became helpless, incontinent, and, soon, died quietly. The longest-staying patient remained 100 days before dying; the shortest was maintained for two weeks and then passed away.

The ages of this group ranged from 19 to 39; four persons were Temne, one was Mende; one man was identified as a "heathen," another man was a "pagan." The religious affiliation of the others was not specified. The occupations of seven of the men included a cook, a trader, a coal heaver, a stoker, a motor apprentice, and two laborers.[3]

MENTAL RETARDATION

Mentally retarded persons were maintained at the asylum from the beginning. Some were distinguished as suffering from "idiotic mania" or "idiocy." Between 1905 and 1925, eight cases, a woman and seven men, received these designations. The youngest of the group was the woman, a 20-year-old trader who came from the Freetown Gaol where she was serving a term for killing her child. She was "physically underdeveloped," had an empty, foolish expression, and, at times, sat for hours "doing nothing but laughing at herself."

The oldest of the group was a 40-year-old farmer who had "a general appearance of a mental degenerate" and was "irrational and stupid." When excited, the chief of his village reported, he attacked others. The reason for his institutionalization, however, was his total inability to care for himself. In the hospital, he remained mute and unresponsive, and passed urine and feces without notice.

The other cases also created trouble and could not care for themselves. This behavior was displayed in public or in the privacy of a home. A 34-year-old man, for example, was taken from the streets where he was "wandering aimlessly" and "throwing stones at people." A 36-year-old Aku farmer created so much disturbance at home that his wife called for his incarceration at Kissy.

Whatever the cause for admission, in every instance, these individuals were described as being "silly and stupid," or having "a vacant, stupid appearance," or "a vacant expression." Only one of these patients returned home. The others died in the asylum, some after developing severe diarrhea, which left them prostrated and emaciated. Ethnically this was a diverse group, composed of two Limba, an Aku (Krio), a Syrian, a Mende, and a Sherbro. Six persons had previous occupations: two farmers, two laborers, and two traders.[4]

Forty-seven additional patients, thirty-eight male and nine female, admitted to the asylum between 1905 and 1959, may also be placed in the category of mentally retarded. While a specific label was not given to these individuals, the notations on each case identified the problem clearly. For example, the varied remarks to designate them include "clearly of low intelligence," "very low mentality," "imbecile of low mentality," "greatly retarded mentally," "feeble-minded,""simple-minded and an idiot," "obviously mentally defective,""mentally deficient," "deficient mental development," and "feeble intellect."

Five of this group stayed in the hospital for less than one month; they were discharged either to relatives or to a tribal ruler in Freetown. One man absconded; one woman went to a female infirmary; three other patients were sent to King George VI Memorial Home, a facility for the homeless located a short distance from the asylum. The remaining cases were maintained at the institution for years. A few were eventually discharged to relatives, but most of them died in the asylum. The longest period of residence was thirty-nine years.

One child was in this group, a 13-year-old boy who was sent home after two years of institutionalization. Aside from this youngster, the group included a wide spread of ages, ranging from 18 to 60. The major ethnic groups of the country were still represented. While some gave no designation, the group that did included fifteen Temne, four Mende, three Limba, three Foulah, three Creole (Krio), three Liberated African Descendant (Krio), a Sierra Leonean (Krio), two Sherbro, and one each of the following: Kroo, Susu, Loko, Kono, Congo, and Mandingo. Most of the members of the group received no occupational specification; the few who were identified included four laborers, two farmers, two fishermen, a pauper, two traders, and four prisoners. The character of the mentally retarded patients was consistently described as being dull, backward, and dependent; some, however, did become violent and destructive.[5]

EPILEPSY

Numerous cases of epilepsy were accommodated at Kissy. This disorder aroused anxiety; many Africans believed that an epileptic fit signified that a sinister, malevolent force, a devil, was struggling within an individual's body. To thwart this evil and prevent contamination, no one dared touch a person during and after an attack. In effect, a grand mal seizure was viewed as a personal threat rather than as evidence of a disorder or sickness requiring the attention of a physician. While this belief mitigated against medical treatment of an afflicted person, the generally perceived frightening nature of the disorder encouraged incarceration. Isolating an epileptic in an institution removed a threat to the community.

Between 1905 and 1959, seventy-eight cases of epilepsy, thirteen female and sixty-five male, were admitted to the asylum. Twenty-two persons, three female and nineteen male, were specifically labeled epileptics, suffering from "epileptic mania." The rest were nondesignated epileptic cases.

In the designated group, one of the women went to an infirmary and the other two women died a few days after admission. A 68-year-old woman, for example, suffered "46 fits" in one evening, followed by "32 fits" the next day. She was brought to the asylum on a stretcher, and, after experiencing repeated attacks, died of exhaustion. Only two of the designated male epileptics were released: a 20-year-old was discharged to the care of his friends and an 18-year-old went to an infirmary. The remaining male patients in this group died in the institution: eleven in less than six months, one after eight months, one after a year, and four after six years.

While many of these patients arrived in a weak, emaciated condition, others followed a basic pattern of behavior. After committing some public disturbance, they were physically restrained by police escorts and brought to the asylum. A 35-year-old laborer, for example, accosted and obstructed passers-by in the streets. Soon after his admission, he had "12 seizures," remained unconscious, sank to a semicomatose state, and, in a few days, died of "epileptic exhaustion." After breaking into a house and damaging property, a 40-year-old man was sent to the asylum, where he had several seizures and in three days died of exhaustion. A 50-year-old farmer, who walked about naked and attacked people in the streets, had a series of "fits" at Kissy, and he, too, died of exhaustion. Six of the male cases came from the Freetown Gaol, where they had displayed violent behavior, striking other people without provocation.

Wherever the scene of the attacks, the prison or the streets, the methods used to control belligerency and seizures remained the same: the disturbed person was isolated in a cell and given a sedative. Such measures facilitated the management of difficult persons, but the deteriorating nature and course of their disorder was not altered.

In the nondesignated group, all of the fifty-six patients were obviously severe cases. Their characteristics were essentially the same as those persons labeled as epileptics. Four were brought to the asylum in a very wasted physical condition: one was partially paralyzed and unable to walk, and the others could not care for themselves, refusing food and medication. In a few days, after having a series of attacks, they died.

The other remaining persons in this group, before being admitted to the asylum, had exhibited threatening behavior or committed an act of violence. They were described as "menacing," "fierce," "exceedingly troublesome," or "dangerous to others." More specifically, a 35-year-old housewife attacked her daughter with stones, a 21-year-old man prevented people from walking in the streets, a 26-year-old woman set a house on fire, a 40-year-old man assaulted people without provocation, and a 36-year-old woman ran in front of moving vehicles, trying to stop them. Others started fights, destroyed property, or chased children.

Invariably, after admission to Kissy, the patients experienced frequent and intense seizures. Seventeen inmates did gain sufficient health and well-being to be discharged, five were released into the community, five were assigned to the care of relatives, three returned to prison, and four, somewhat physically incapacitated, were sent to infirmaries. Thirty-one other patients died in the asylum; eighteen within one year, the rest after periods of residence ranging from one to thirteen years. Clearly, many of these cases were among the most difficult and violent, as well as untreatable, patients admitted to the institution.

Other demographic information further characterizes these groups. Of the seventy-eight designated and nondesignated epilepsy cases, fifty-eight had an ethnic identification. This group included nineteen Mende, ten Temne, one Kono, two Kroo, one Limba, four Sierra Leoneans (Krio), four Aku (Krio), five Creole (Krio), one Liberated African Descendant (Krio), one Liberian, one Spanish, two Mandingo, two Gambian, one Nigerian, two Eboe, and one Hausa. Forty-nine from these groups, five women and forty-four men, received an occupational designation. Among the women, there were two traders, two nurses, and a housewife. The men included a cook, three laborers, a goldsmith, a stonemason, fourteen farmers, a fisherman, a writing clerk, an evangelist, two shoemakers, three traders, a solder, a painter, and fourteen prisoners. Prior to 1916, the religion of each patient was often specified; fifteen epileptics received a religious label, and included one "Mohamedan," two "Heathen," five "Pagan," three Protestant, and four Christian. The ages of these clients ranged from 18 to 68, with the majority of them in their twenties and thirties.[6]

ALCOHOLISM AND DRUG ADDICTION

During the colonial era, mental illnesses related to alcohol consumption and drug addiction remained a minor concern. Until the 1920s, only one case of alcoholic psychosis, labeled "alcoholic mania" is recorded. This was a 42-year-old man, an Aku, who was identified as suicidal by police and taken to the asylum in February 1909. While occasionally he demanded whiskey, his condition remained unchanged for years. He kept to himself, engaged in random incoherent conversation, took food well, assisted in work details, and eventually, in April 1925, was discharged to the care of his sister.[7]

Between 1925 and 1959, the case books identify thirteen other persons, twelve men and a woman, with maladies involving intoxicating beverages. Only one man was a long-term case, a 32-year-old African sailor. He was viewed as suffering from alcoholic psychosis and tagged "an unrepented alcoholic" who, though seemingly quiet and rational, became at times excitable and aggressive. At night, he heard "singing in the breeze," and for hours, in response, he sang along. He remained at Kissy for twenty years. The only woman in this group, a 35-year-old Temne, confessed to being intoxicated before she was admitted to the asylum, and eventually, after nearly two years, she proved unable to care for herself and was transferred to an infirmary. A man, a 23-year-old Kissi driver, became ill after consuming too much wine; he went to the hospital and became violent. One week later he was discharged, and he never returned to the asylum.

The other cases were similar instances of heavy drinking followed by scenes of disorderly conduct and violence. The offenders were incarcerated for short periods of time and then released. Three men compiled histories of "heavy drinking" and were readmitted at a later date. The ethnic makeup of these alcoholics included three Temne, a Mende, an Eboe, a Loko, a Limba, a Kissi, a Syrian, and two Africans (Krio). Their ages were largely in the twenties and thirties with one 50-year-old man.[8]

Drug addiction, notably the smoking of *Cannabis sativa* or marijuana, appeared in these years and frequently, according to the case records, caused violent and bizarre behavior. Sixteen drug cases, all males and most in their late twenties, were taken to Kissy for observation. The ethnic sample included eight

Temne, one Mende, one Koranko, one Bassa, one Gambian, and two Gold Coastians. In almost every case, the person's smoking of marijuana produced aggressive, intolerable acts. For example, a 28-year-old Temne farmer flogged his wife and tore his clothes; another Temne farmer, a 34-year-old man, set fire to a house; a 28-year-old Koranko laborer fought in the streets. Seven men from this group were prisoners. Under the influence of marijuana they had become belligerent and started fights in the jail or had engaged in such unsavory acts as smearing feces over themselves and cell walls, which led to their transfer to the mental hospital. Only one of the addicts became a long-term patient - a 20-year-old Mende farmer who, after being maintained at the institution for twenty years, was discharged to the care of his brothers. The majority of drug patients were short-term inmates who were discharged after residing in the hospital for a few weeks.[9]

This basic policy was confirmed by M.C.F. Easmon, the African physician and specialist on mental disorders at the Kissy asylum, who noted in a December 1920 memo how addiction affected behavior. His subject was a 26-year-old male trader who was noisy and dangerous and often howled and rolled on the ground. Easmon commented: "I have just found out that he is in the habit of smoking "jamba," a local cannabis...which produces temporary mania. I have had several cases at Kissy in recent years." Easmon maintained that this mental condition was transitory, and that after a few days or weeks, a marijuana patient recovered and could be discharged.[10]

While Easmon's remarks suggest that some drug dependency may not have been recorded, the small number of users entering Kissy asylum at this time contrasts with the deluge of drug consumers that emerged in much later years. In the period after 1960, drug addiction in Sierra Leone became increasingly a social and mental health problem, as revealed in the rapid growth of crime and delinquency and related sociopathic problems.

GENERAL PARALYSIS OF THE INSANE

General paralysis of the insane, or GPI, a psychiatric designation used widely in American and British mental hospitals in the early twentieth century, was applied to mental patients in Sierra Leone. Over time, as noted earlier, GPI was more precisely diagnosed as tertiary syphilis. Between 1905 and 1945, sixty-three persons at Kissy were identified with this malady - five women and fifty-eight men. These individuals had a relatively short stay in the institution: six were discharged within a month, four went to an infirmary, and two were sent to relatives or friends. All of the other GPI patients died, as expected, in the institution - fifty-one in less than a year. Of that number, thirty-five expired in less than ninety days.

The average age of the GPI patient was 45, a fairly advanced time of life for early-twentieth-century Africa but characteristic of the disease. Ethnically, this largely middle-aged group embraced nine Temne, nine Mende, five Aku (Krio), two Sierra Leoneans (Krio), two Creole (Krio), one Liberated African Descendant (Krio), three Limba, one Portuguese, one Loko, three Kroo, one Bassa, one Susu, a Yoruba, a Jollof, a Liberian, a Gambian, a West Indian, and a Jamaican. Only a few patients were linked to a religion or a religious denomination: two "Mohamedan," two Church of England, three Protestant, three Christian, and one Wesleyan.

A sample of the occupational standing of the GPI group included the following: three prisoners, eight farmers, three sailors, a washerman, six fishermen, four laborers, a painter, a stonemason, a goldsmith, a writing clerk, a pensioner, a blacksmith, a cook, two watchmen, a carpenter, two soldiers, a dresser, and a trader. Two of the female GPI patients were traders.[11]

GPI patients usually arrived at the institution in a weak, almost emaciated condition. Several inmates were found "wandering about aimlessly" in the streets; nearly all of them were labeled "incoherent" and were unable to answer questions in a rational manner. Some were said to look dazed or confused, or had a "general demented appearance" and were incapable of caring for themselves. Others threatened violence, or actually had destroyed property or attacked persons. In some instances, there were obvious indications of physical debility: a patient "walks about staggering," or "can't stand or walk without difficulty," or "trembled when moved," or was "unable to sit up or remain seated." Some suffered from "partial paralysis," or "paralysis of the muscles." These were typical signs of nervous system syphilis.

Soon after admission to the asylum, in a few days or weeks, GPI patients not already disabled became weak and feeble and could not walk. The physical degeneration became obvious; the case records document how inmates were "losing flesh daily." A stimulant - milk and brandy or ferri tonic - was administered, but invariably did not improve the increasingly helpless and moribund condition of the afflicted.

The notations of the final hours of a 45-year-old man illustrate the difficult, irreversible nature of the disorder: "every four hours condition weaker. cannot speak audibly. getting prostrated. semi-unconsciousness toward evening. toward dawn condition changed for the worse. unconsciousness deepened. despite all attendance, patient died at 6 AM." Another patient, a 48-year-old Mende fisherman, prostrated and defenseless, was found at night swarmed by driver ants. The ants completely covered him, "some entering his mouth, ears, and nostrils." Reduced to this state, he became enveloped in a profound unconsciousness and was unable to take food or medication; he soon wasted away and died. His death attributed to general paralysis of the insane, albeit accelerated by the bites of driver ants.

MELANCHOLIA

Between 1905 and 1959, melancholia, another standard turn-of-the century psychiatric designation, was applied to sixty-nine mental patients - twenty-three female and forty-six male - at the Kissy asylum. Those melancholics assuming an ethnic identity included two Sierra Leoneans (Krio), four Aku (Krio), two Creole (Krio), one African (Krio), one Kroo, three Limba, eight Mende, eight Temne, one Sherbro, two Foulah, and one from each of the following groups: Loko, Gambian, Popo, Calabar, Hausa, Yoruba, Lagosian, Jamaican, Indian, German.

Occupations of the male members of the group included a steward, two tailors, two laborers, four clerks, three farmers, a drum beater, a soldier, two traders, four prisoners, two carpenters, and a police sergeant; among the females, there were a marketwoman, a schoolteacher, and two traders.

The ages of the group ranged largely over the twenties and thirties but with a significant gender distinction: of the thirty-one males who specified their ages, fifteen were under the age of 30 and eleven were above 40; of the twenty females who gave their age, only one was under 30 and nine were over 40. These figures suggest that melancholia affected females at a later time in life than males.

Many of the melancholics remained in the institution for a long period of time: thirty-three resided in the hospital for over one year. Of these, thirteen women and seven men died in the facility, one woman after twenty-six years of hospitalization and a man after thirty-one years of institutional life. Twelve other patients, two women and ten men, died in the asylum after less than one year's residence. Only eleven melancholics were short-term inmates: eight men and three women were discharged in less than thirty days. The remaining thirteen patients, four women and nine men, left the hospital after periods of stay ranging from two months to a year.

Melancholics, like other mentally distressed persons, were brought to the asylum for disturbing the peace, being troublesome at home, or for acting in a foolish manner and not being able to account for themselves. In many instances, however, they displayed other kinds of behavior. As was typical of melancholic patients everywhere, a suicidal tendency was evident: a Nigerian man tried to cut his throat, a 30-year-old woman threatened to kill herself and her child, and a 22-year-old man, a Mende farmer, was admitted with self-inflicted knife wounds. Several from the group seemed lost and abandoned, as well as detached from their surroundings. One man was found lying in the street in a helpless condition; another man was "aimlessly wandering about town" picking up waste paper. Others loitered in the streets, near public buildings, oblivious to traffic and people.

In the hospital, these patients displayed the classic outward signs of this disorder. Case records observed that the individual "sits in a melancholic condition," or has "sudden fits of depression"; patients were said to have "a depressed melancholy look," or "a melancholic appearance," or "in a condition of lugubrious melancholy," or "depressed in mind."

Most melancholics were dependent and nonviolent and remained quiet, listless, sad, and morose, taking no interest in anything or anyone. Over time, however, some did gain enough composure to help in the kitchen, with the laundry, or to assist in yard work or some other work detail. The general condition of the long-term melancholic remained unchanged: this person was "noisy at times," but typically was silent, took food well, and gave no trouble - a pattern broken only by some physical disorder that contributed to the patient's death.

After World War II, the designation "melancholy" was used infrequently; it was replaced by the term "depression." Most patients were not assigned to any specific depressive disorders. Instead, the notations in the casebooks refer occasionally to inmates who had "a fixed depressed look," or were simply "depressed" or "very depressed."[12]

SUICIDE

During the twentieth century colonial period in Sierra Leone, fifty-nine cases - seventeen females and forty-two males - relating to suicide were admitted to the Kissy asylum. Five additional patients, a woman and four men, were melancholics. These numbers reflect a basic trend: suicide appears to be a minor problem in African society. Certain factors may act as deterrents: a sense of personal guilt is absent from traditional African culture, and strong taboos militate against suicide. A family is shamed by a person's self-destruction; in some areas, it has jeopardized an inheritance. Many believe that suicide is a contagious evil. The body of a suicide is buried quickly and without a ceremony. If a person hanged himself in a tree, that tree is cut down and burnt; the house in which an individual killed himself is destroyed and abandoned.[13]

All of the fifty-nine cases at Kissy represented attempted suicide, or parasuicide. The majority of the members of this group were above 40 years of age and were nondesignated psychiatric cases. Twelve male suicidals received a diagnosis. These diagnoses included one acute dementia, two senile dementia, one dementia, one schizophrenia paranoid, one delusional insanity, one subacute mania, three acute mania, one GPI, and one alcoholic mania. Forty-seven remained without a psychiatric identification. Over half of these patients left the facility within eight months; the others resided in the asylum for periods ranging from one year to thirty-four years. The ethnic breakdown of suicide cases embraced fifteen Mende, a Temne, six Aku (Krio), a Creole (Krio), a Sierra Leonean (Krio), five Kroo, one Foulah, two Syrian, a Limba, two Susu, and a Yoruba.

In most instances, the reasons given for the parasuicide were vague. For example, the records of a prisoner sent to Kissy specify that he had "a suicidal tendency." Others had "a suicidal intent," some felt depressed and tried self-destruction, and some had simply "attempted suicide." A few cases were more explicit: a 45-year-old Foulah said a devil made him stab himself. A 24-year-old Mende man, fearing a beating, decided "to die for myself" and jumped into an open well. Another man, claiming that he was "bewitched," tried to drown himself and, later, placed himself across a railroad track. A woman, lamenting the death of her child, also stretched herself across a railroad bed.

Another woman cut into her abdomen, believing that something was "eating her up inside."

The dread or fear of disease, namely pneumonia, gonorrhea, and syphilis, accounted for three attempted suicides. Some of the methods of self-destruction included hanging, drinking poison, cutting wrists or throat, jumping from a high place, leaping from a train, plunging over a sea wall, and springing in front of a moving car or train.[14]

MANIA

Over the years 1905 to 1959, large groups of patients were placed in the acute and chronic mania categories. The number of acute mania cases stood at 143, including 41 women and 102 men. Most of these persons died in the institution; only thirty-three individuals were returned to the community. The majority of deaths and discharges occurred during the first year of hospitalization: seventeen women and fifty-two men died, while five women and twenty-one men were discharged. Within five years of institutionalization, fifteen additional male acute mania patients died, and six were discharged; and seven female patients died and two were discharged. Among the long-term cases, fourteen remained over five years. The longest-staying male died after eighteen years, while the oldest female acute maniac died after thirty years of asylum care.

A significant age difference distinguished male and female acute maniacs. The males were younger than the females: while the ages ranged from 14 to 60 years for males and from 20 to 60 for the females, most of the males were in their late twenties and early thirties and the females in their late thirties and early forties.

The ethnic mix of the group included thirty-five Mende, fourteen Temne, eleven Sierra Leoneans (Krio), one African (Krio), two Liberated African Descendant (Krio), four Aku (Krio), one Creole (Krio), five Limba, five Kroo, five Susu, three Loko, three Sherbro, one Koranko, two Foulah, two Yoruba, one Eboe, four Mandingo, three Gambian, two West Indian, one Jamaican, one Indian, one Syrian, one Congo, and one Chinese.

The occupations of the acute maniacs were, for the females, nine traders, a seamstress, a laborer, a laundress, a farmer, and a prisoner. The male patients' occupations were as follows: twenty-one farmers, seventeen laborers, ten prisoners, nine soldiers, four carpenters, three fishermen, two traders, two goldsmiths, two seamen, two schoolboys, a stonemason, a blacksmith, a policeman, a baker, a shoemaker, a pastor, and a schoolteacher.

Religious affiliations embraced eleven "Pagan," nine "Heathen," ten Christian, five "Mohamedan," one Muslim, four Protestant, two Church of England, one Moravian, one Baptist, three Methodist, one "Infidel," one Wesleyan, and one Greek Orthodox.

The mania cases represented the most violent and destructive types of mental disorder. Whatever the age or the sex, most of these patients were admitted to the asylum because they displayed extreme forms of behavior. The casebooks frequently report some sort of threatening conduct: one person "destroys crops" and "runs after people with a cutlass," another individual "throws stones at people," a man "shouts day and night in the streets, enters private houses and defecates, and threatens to set fire to houses." Another maniac "attempted to bite and injure anyone who came near him"; one individual "wanders about the village making noises and threatening people with a knife"; a man "becomes maniacal on the slightest provocation"; a woman "attacked her old father"; another woman was caught "roaming the streets beating children and passers-by with a stick"; a man had "destroyed other people's property in the marketplace"; one person had "fits of extreme violence"; one individual "suddenly became violent and rushed and jumped through the kitchen window when breakfast was being served." Others simply had "a wild appearance," or "a fugitive and hunted expression," or were brought "in a very violent state," in "a wild condition," or in "a state of wild excitement."

Many came to Kissy under restraint, strapped to a stretcher, wrapped in a hammock, or bound by handcuffs. Much of their violence continued in the institution. Several of the acute maniacs assaulted or fought with other inmates, broke cups and plates, or howled, cried, and sang without stopping for hours. They danced, tore off their clothes and ran about naked, and refused to eat. Individuals displaying such erratic behavior were restrained by a straitjacket or placed in an isolation cell.

Alas, for some patients, only death brought relief. Several days, perhaps weeks, of continued hyperactivity invariably drained a patient, who became thin and emaciated. Efforts at intervention, such as administering a nutrient enema, did not check the patient's deteriorating condition. Numerous patients simply "died of exhaustion following acute mania."[15]

In contrast to the acute maniacs, most of the chronic maniacs were older, more violent, and remained in the institution for a longer time. Thirty-eight persons were designated as chronic maniacs, twenty-two males and sixteen females. From this number, thirty-four died in the asylum, nineteen men and fifteen women; the rest were discharged. Twenty-seven members of the group became long-term residents, staying in the institution for more than one year. One woman died after twenty-one years of hospitalization; one man was released after eight years at Kissy. The majority of the males were in their thirties and forties and most of the females were in their forties.

The major factor for institutionalizing a chronic maniac was an unusual display of violence: one woman, for example, had "uncontrollable fits of violence," another woman "assaulted persons with an axe," still another woman "beats her aged grandmother." A male patient "tried to murder his mother with a machete," another man "attacked his father with a knife," a woman "fights people in the marketplace," a man "sets fire to houses" and "runs into the bush and hides and attacks women and children who pass by."

Some of the chronic maniacs came from the Freetown Gaol, where they had assaulted prisoners or staff, or had demonstrated unruly and unmanageable behavior. As with the acute maniacs, the chronic maniacs remained troublesome in the asylum, necessitating isolation in a special cell or the use of a restraining device to control them.

The ethnic makeup of the group was as follows: three Sierra Leoneans (Krio), three Creole (Krio), three Aku (Krio), three Temne, four Mende, three Eboe, one Yoruba, two Limba, one Kroo, one Sherbro, one Susu, two Mandingo, one Gambian, one Jollof, and one Congo. Occupations for the chronic maniacs were, for the men, five farmers, two laborers, two firemen, a shoeman, a writing clerk, a blacksmith, a fisherman, a carpenter, a stonemason, a schoolmaster, and five prisoners. Among the women, there were a prisoner, six traders, a hawker, a seamstress, and a housemaid. Religious affiliations were five "Pagan," four "Heathen," seven Christian, four Protestant, three "Mohamedan," two Church of England, one Baptist, and one Methodist.[16]

Subacute mania, current mania, recurrent mania, hypomania, mania, maniacal insanity, chronic insanity, and circular insanity were other psychiatric categories used at Kissy before 1960. During this time, twelve cases of subacute mania were designated -

four women and eight men. This was a varied group: the ages stretched from 19 to 66 years, and the periods of residence ranged from fourteen days to eighteen years. Five males died in the asylum, and the remaining cases of subacute mania were discharged. No obvious pattern emerged: one man died after three months of hospitalization, and another man died after eighteen years in the institution; one man was released after fourteen days, and another man spent sixteen years in the facility before being sent back to the community.

The reasons for confinement were varied: while some act of violence or threat of violence was partially responsible for a person's incarceration, other factors recorded on the casebooks include "talks irrationally to self," "doesn't know his whereabouts or past movements," "has no idea of space or time or surroundings," and being "abnormally stubborn," "incoherent in speech," or "more or less helpless."

The subacute mania group included four Mende, two Temne, three Sierra Leoneans (Krio), one Liberated African Descendant (Krio), and one Nigerian. The occupations embraced two farmers, a laborer, a soldier, a pauper, and for the women, a trader and a laundress. The religious affiliations were two "Pagan," two "Heathen," one Christian, and one Protestant.[17]

There were three cases of current mania, two women and a man. One of the women, a 19-year-old laundress from the Gambia, had "outbursts of violence and uncontrollable temper," followed by periods of melancholia. After nearly two years at Kissy, she was discharged. The other woman was 39 years old and had disturbed the peace, throwing stones and bottles at people and saying that she belonged to "a grand society." While she was "very noisy at times," this patient maintained herself, accepting hospital routine and discipline. Over the years, the notations of physicians on her conduct and health were terse and repetitive: "No change noticed in patient's condition," or "Patient going on in the same condition." After thirty-two years in the institution, she died of tuberculosis.

The male "current maniac" was a 32-year-old Temne laborer who had thrown stones at houses and sang and danced at the police station. In the asylum, he was "noisy and violent" and, in six and a half months, he died of tubercular meningitis.[18] A recurrent mania case was a 47-year-old Krio housewife, a quarrelsome, destructive, agitated person who died after six years of institutionalization.[19]

There were four hypomania cases, three men and a woman. The female, a Temne, remained at Kissy for over twenty-three years, suffering from Parkinson's disease. One of the men, a 29-year-old Susu, was found shouting in a law court, and he also died after twenty-three years in the asylum. Another man, a 40-year-old Mende, was released to a relative who promised to care for him. The fourth hypomania case was a 28-year-old Temne trader who, because of his violent, aggressive nature, was kept isolated for much of the time. After eight and a half years of residence, he died in the asylum.[20]

One case of undifferentiated mania is recorded, a 35-year-old Mende man who had "vacant looks," walked about aimlessly at night, and drank his own urine. He died of "general debility" after twenty-three days in the hospital.[21] A Krio laundress suffered from "maniacal insanity," and after twelve days at Kissy was discharged to the care of her relatives.[22] Also, a 39-year-old man was specified as suffering from "chronic insanity." He molested people in the streets, was "excited" and "noisy," and saw things others did not see. Ten months after his admission, he died of ascites.[23]

The label "circular insanity" was given to a 22-year-old man who was violent and incoherent; supposedly he could laugh, cry, and whistle simultaneously. He spent a month in the asylum and was discharged to the care of his brother.[24] Another psychiatric identification, "confusional insanity," was attributed to four men. A 60-year-old Limba man, associated with "irresponsible action" and irrational conversation, spent six weeks in the asylum before being sent to an infirmary. The other three confusional cases were also disoriented and could not care for themselves; they died in the institution.[25]

DEMENTIA

Some patients were placed in the categories of acute dementia, dementia, senile dementia, chronic dementia, and primary dementia. For example, acute dementia was applied to a 35-year-old man from the Gold Coast who showed no interest in himself or his surroundings. At times, he was "very noisy," shouting and fighting with other inmates; often, he sat by himself and refused to work. Over time, he became a shadowy figure. His case record notes: "There is nothing to report about him." After twelve years of hospitalization, he died of heart failure and mitral valve disease.[26]

Eleven patients, five female and six male, were designated as sufferers of dementia. Unable to care for themselves, they could not accept discipline and annoyed other inmates. Two dementia cases, a 36-year-old man and a 40-year-old man, were discharged; the others either died in the hospital or were transferred, in a physically weak condition, to an infirmary.

The dementia cases included two Temne, one Mende, one Mandingo, and one Sherbro. Occupationally, there were a prisoner, two farmers, a laborer, and a shopboy.[27]

Nine senile dementia patients, four female and five male, were identified. This group comprised two Mende, two Sierra Leoneans (Krio), one Liberated African Descendant (Krio), one African (Krio), one Mandingo, one Foulah, and one Yoruba. Four males were discharged to relatives or to an infirmary; the other senile cases passed away in the asylum. Each was of an advanced age and in a totally dependent, run-down, feeble condition: death was attributed to senile dementia as a primary cause.[28]

There were two chronic dementia cases: a Mende man labeled "a destitute and a public nuisance" who was transferred to an infirmary, and a 40-year-old Temne farmer, a confused, anxious, talkative man who, after three months, died of heart and kidney failure.[29]

Thirteen primary dementia patients were identified, seven women and six men. Four were discharged, and the nine remaining persons died in the institution. The members of this group were younger than those in other dementia categories; six of the seven women, for example, were under 40. The primary dementia inmates displayed behavior typical of the conduct of persons being sent to Kissy. They were "troublesome," or "incoherent," or "aggressive"; some had attacked people in the streets. The ethnic ties of this group embraced five Mende, one Temne, two Creole (Krio), two Sierra Leoneans (Krio), one Sherbro, and one Loko.[30]

SCHIZOPHRENIA

Beginning in the early 1940s, schizophrenia increasingly became a psychiatric category applied to patients at Kissy Mental Hospital. Dementia praecox, the early-twentieth century term for schizophrenia, was specified for three inmates: a 20-year-old violent but physically debilitated Temne man who died uncertified six days after being admitted; a 36-year-old "bewitched" Yoruba fisherman who was institutionalized for six years; and a 30-year-old Kroo man, a person who did not want to leave the asylum, but was sent, eventually, after four years and nine months, to an infirmary.[31]

There were forty-eight cases labeled schizophrenia - thirty-five male and thirteen female. They were broken down into four groups: eighteen schizophrenia, twelve male and six female; twenty-one schizophrenia paranoid type, fifteen male and six female; eight schizophrenia simple type, six male and two female; and one male schizophrenia hebephrenic type.

The ethnic makeup of these groupings embraced eleven Mende, eight Temne, ten Creole (Krio), two Sierra Leoneans (Krio), two Foulah, two Kroo, one Limba, one Sherbro, one Susu, one Kono, one Hausa, one Gambian, and one Jollof. The ages of the schizophrenics stretched from 22 to 52; the majority of the males were in their twenties and thirties, the females in their thirties and forties.

The most enduring and obvious characteristic of the schizophrenics was long-term institutionalization. Only six of the forty-eight patients were discharged after a short stay in the asylum. The remaining schizophrenics became truly the incurables, the chronic insane. Their length of hospitalization averaged over ten years, and eight patients remained over twenty years. Many died in the institution, and others were sent to King George VI Memorial Home.

Most patients adjusted to asylum life. In some instances, however, an inmate's behavior deteriorated: a Mende woman, for example, after seven years in the asylum, became withdrawn and developed catatonic features; another female patient became suspicious and inaccessible. But most of the schizophrenic cases stayed basically the same, showing no improvement or regression. A man who resided at the hospital for eleven years displayed "no real change in his mental state." He was described as "well institutionalized." A laborer, after six years of hospital life, continued to be "oblivious to his surroundings."

Many inmates received "no visitors" and gave "no trouble"; only the manner of their death broke the hospital routine. After twenty-one years in the asylum, an inmate died, not knowing where he had been. "It was reported that the patient was found dead on the floor at 11 PM last night." Over the years, most of these patients kept physically healthy. While they stayed in a "satisfactory condition" or "good physical condition," their thought processes and actions were characterized as "mostly paranoid and deluded," "delusive and irresponsible," or "confused and irrelevant." They did acquire sufficient control to par-

ticipate in a work routine; a few were called "good workers."
Some were transferred to the memorial home. A 50-year-old
Mende woman, for example, was called "a cheerful old thing,"
and after seven years at the hospital was declared "suitable" for
discharge to the institution of the homeless.

In effect, these schizophrenics had become totally dependent on
an institution. They had traits common to long-term patients at
mental hospitals in other parts of the world, developing a condition called hospitalism or institutionalism or "institutional
neurosis." This was a pattern of behavior distinguished by
apathy, no interest in the future, deterioration of personal habits,
resigned acceptance of and submission to institutional rules, and
an inability to imagine a life outside of the hospital.[32]

DELUSIONS

Between 1905 and 1959, delusional insanity was assigned to
forty-three patients - four women and thirty-nine men. This
group consisted largely of middle-aged persons, with five inmates
under 32, and a 61-year-old man. While sixteen patients died in
the hospital, fourteen others were discharged in less than a year,
and four individuals stayed at Kissy for more than ten years. The
ethnic breakdown of the group included eleven Temne, five
Mende, five Sierra Leoneans (Krio), three Aku (Krio), one
Liberated African Descendant (Krio), six Sherbro, three Susu,
one Calabar, and one Kissi.

Some of the delusions lacked specificity: one person was
"dazed" and "delusional"; another "suffered from hallucinations"
and felt "bewitched"; two others succumbed simply to
"delusional insanity." On the other hand, some delusions were
quite vivid and concrete: a 35-year-old man had a serpent in his
ear who talked to him; a 42-year-old Mende butcher had "delusions of grandeur," asserting that he owned the asylum, the railroad, the prisons, and all the cows of Sierra Leone. He also
claimed to control the government and said he was president of
the United States. A 35-year-old Mende man said that he had
bought the world, was "general manager" of England, and
wanted to arrest seven thousand people. A 23-year-old man made
claims to property that was owned by others, and a 45-year-old
Aku stonemason charged that the government and a French company owed him "plenty money." This was an unfortunate case: a
medical officer commented that he was a harmless person and "it

seems a pity to certify" him insane. Alas, no one could be found to care for him, and he remained in the institution for over twenty-two years.[33]

Many other patients at the Kissy asylum, without being assigned to any psychiatric category, also held delusions and a noticeable number related to money, property, and positions of power. Some of these persons stated simply that they had "much money," or "large sums of money," or "money hidden." One man said he had six million pounds; a 49-year-old Aku writing clerk claimed that the government of Sierra Leone had stolen the money sent to him by the King of England; a 35-year-old Kroo man insisted that he had received a large sum of money from the Bank of England but had lost his bank book, and, consequently, could not receive the money. One man lamented that he had left his wealth on board several ships and said that it would "fill the asylum building." Another asserted that he had "wealth, property, and several wives."

Delusions about being a powerful person figured prominently in the inner world of several patients. Some inmates assumed the identity of a paramount chief. Others simulated more powerful positions: a man said that he was "King of Sierra Leone," a 27-year-old Temne man claimed himself "King of England," a 39-year-old writing clerk was "King of all Africans," a 46-year-old man believed that he was "King of the World," and a Krio man called himself "Imperial Earl of Ireland." A 32-year-old man, who was "not in touch with reality," said his father was the American president, Franklin D. Roosevelt. One woman, characterized as "abusive and incoherent," was a "Queen," a 35-year-old Mende woman claimed that the Mende God was her husband.[34]

Numerous patients were affected by religious delusions. Three cases were specifically labeled religious mania. In February 1911, the police brought to the asylum a 41-year-old man who had been preaching and shouting in the streets. He continued preaching in the hospital, usually about four times a day, remained nonviolent, disturbed no one, and died quietly of heart failure in September 1913. Another instance of religious mania involved a 26-year-old man who viewed himself as a prophet, claiming that God had placed "a sun in his head." He was hospitalized for a few weeks until relatives agreed to take care of him. The third case of religious mania was a 34-year-old man identified as a Mandingo preacher who wandered about the colony and the protectorate calling himself a prophet. Incarcerated at Kissy in August 1922, he died in the institution eight years later.[35]

Forty-one other patients, ten women and thirty-one men, not specifically labeled religious maniacs, were nonetheless afflicted by delusions of a religious nature. Five of the men, and a 55-year-old Krio housewife, each claimed to be God. A Kroo housewife said she "used to be God," a 23-year-old Krio man saw himself as the "Lord of Creation," a 32-year-old shoemaker was the "son of God," and four inmates said that they had been "sent by God." One woman was noted as a "religious fanatic," suffering from "religious exaltation"; she was noisy, singing and preaching at night, and she talked all day about "things pertaining to religion." Another man had a fixed delusion that he was the angel Gabriel. He wore feathers in his ear, claiming that the plumage came from the wings of an angel. He also asserted that the morning mist was "the smoke of people burning in Hell" and that the Holy Ghost had made all the marks on his body.

As a group, these inmates were middle-aged. Twenty-two died in the hospital, and the remainder were released to relatives or sent to the memorial home. They were nonviolent but became boisterous, sermonizing frequently in lengthy harangues at irregular hours of the day and night.[36]

WITCHCRAFT

A belief in witches and devils was held by some clients of the Kissy asylum. Witchcraft permeated traditional African life surreptitiously. It represented an umbrella concept covering all forms of supernatural authority that bring trouble, and occasionally healing, to its victims. Experiences of misfortune were especially attributed to the influence of witchcraft. Such events might include sickness, business failure, rejection by a spouse or lover, and almost any sort of loss or defeat. A person might fancy himself bewitched after experiencing a witchcraft dream or nightmare. And many people accepted a direct connection between witchcraft and mental illness, believing that madness was simply a concrete manifestation of some evil power over the demented person. In effect, it was believed that witchcraft caused bizarre or abnormal behavior, demonstrating dramatically its ability to dominate an individual.

At Kissy Mental Hospital between 1905 and 1959, 145 patients - 112 men and 33 women - made specific reference to witchcraft. The largest number of this group, 103 individuals, were nondesignated cases. The designated cases included the following:

one subacute mania, eleven acute mania, three melancholia, two GPI, one alcoholic mania, six epileptic, one hypomania, one schizophrenia paranoid, two primary dementia, and one mentally retarded.

The ethnic groupings embraced thirty-six Temne, twenty-five Mende, ten Sierra Leonean (Krio), seven Aku (Krio), seven Creole (Krio), two African (Krio), one Liberated African Descendant (Krio), three Foulah, two Yoruba, one Loko, two Bassa, three Limba, two Jollof, one Mandingo, three Susu, one Kroo, one Gambian, one Hausa, four Kono, three Kissi, one Koranko, one Sherbro, and one Lagosian. No special age characterized this group; the majority of the men and women were in their twenties, thirties, and forties.

Some of these individuals just saw "devils," beings who took the form of shadowy amorphous figures, representing a threatening force. With different individuals, the devil could be a man or woman, black or white. For other persons, however, the devil or devils acquired unique characteristics. One man envisioned the devil as a leopard; a 35-year-old Krio woman saw devils, "sometimes with no head, sometimes with four heads"; a 20-year-old woman observed a devil "resembling a dog with chicken eyes which followed her about"; and a 47-year-old Jollof man viewed a devil "with 65 feet who persuaded him to make presents to children."

A devil could remain with a person over a long time period: a 26-year-old Mende soldier, for example, asserted that "a white woman devil" came to him when he was ten years old, requesting that he follow her. She went away when his father tied "medicine" around his waist. Later, away from home and in the army, the "medicine" was no longer available, and the woman devil returned, asking him to marry her. He refused, saying that others had to consent, and she gave him a cup of coffee that made him choke. This woman appeared frequently, most often at night, to play with him, always demanding that he run away with her.

On occasion, patients assumed the role of an evil-doer: one man said that he was the devil, implying that he was the source of evil; another man stated that "a devil came to him and made him invulnerable," giving him the power to harm others with impunity. A 35-year-old woman, calling herself God, asserted that she had killed several persons by witchcraft; another woman also claimed that witchcraft had allowed her to kill people. A 30-year-old washerwoman maintained that a devil gave her the "powers of sorcery," permitting her to transform a person into a lower animal. On the other hand, two women declared themselves innocent of witchcraft, alleging that they had been abused and attacked by people who had named them witches.

Several patients believed themselves bewitched, possessed, or troubled by witches. A 28-year-old Kissi man confessed to being "possessed by a black female devil." In some instances, the actual physical presence of a witch or devil seemed most apparent to a person. A man was convinced that a devil "holds him"; another man insisted that devils "play with him when he is lying down." A Temne woman said that a devil was inside her head; another complained of "three little devils in one ear and two in another." A 34-year-old Temne prisoner believed that devils were "interfering with the workings of his internal organs."

In a few cases, a devil brought health and wealth. While a Temne woman believed that her devil brought her food and rice, a Temne man said his devil would meet him in Freetown and give him medicine that would cure him. A 43-year-old Temne prisoner held a delusion that his devil gave him money and a large house. However, in most instances, a devil brought pain, frequently a headache, and caused improper conduct. A 30-year-old Mende soldier claimed a devil attacked him in his sleep, making him fight others. A 38-year-old prisoner charged that "a devil with many heads" intimidated him and caused his outbursts of wild behavior.

Several inmates attributed their mental suffering to a devil. Most of these patients remained anxious and full of dread. Terrorized by apparent devils, they anticipated and feared attacks and mortal combat. A few took protective measures. To ward off witches, a woman rubbed dirt and charcoal on her face; a man demanded "a piece of charcoal to chew and swallow" in order to get rid of a serpent and a devil that were inside of him; a 30-year-old farmer requested "a pure white sheep" to sacrifice and to "make a feast to banish his devil." A 24-year-old Mende steward intended to "buy sheep to give to his devil." And a 45-year-old Mende farmer began every morning of his residence at the asylum by shouting curses at his enemies "for three hours at a stretch," in an effort to fend off evil powers.[37]

NON-DESIGNATED CASES

Between 1905 and 1959, 1,716 persons - 1,262 men and 454 women - entered Kissy Mental Hospital as nondesignated cases, and they remained unclassified regardless of the length of hospital residence. This was largely a middle-aged group. While the men ranged in age from 14 to 80 and the women from 18 to 78, the males averaged in their mid-thirties, and the females in their early forties. From this group, 733 patients were discharged or died within a month of admission; over 200 left within a year; 46 were returned to prison; and 301 remained in the hospital for more than one year. The longest hospital stays were thirty-four years for a male, and twenty-eight years for a female. Three hundred and fifty of the discharged inmates were sent to an infirmary at Kissy, a place previously known as the incurable hospital; later this facility was phased out and its clientele joined the homeless and the debilitated or incapacitated inmates at King George VI Memorial Home.

The ethnic groups of the nondesignated patients included: 288 Temne, 214 Mende, 112 Sierra Leonean (Krio), 65 Creole (Krio), 48 Aku (Krio), 18 Liberated African Descendant (Krio), 31 African (Krio), 65 Limba, 64 Kroo, 56 Susu, 43 Loko, 40 Mandingo, 37 Foulah, 22 Sherbro, 16 Kissi, 13 Kono, 13 Koranko, 10 Yoruba, 10 Eboe, 10 Jollof, 7 Fanti, 6 Syrian, 6 Gambian, 5 Nigerian, 5 Hausa, 3 Gold Coastian, 3 Liberian, 3 West Indian, 2 European, 2 Sengalese, 2 Jamaican, 2 Lagosian, 1 Chinese, 1 Indian, 1 Yolunka, 1 Accra, 1 Congo, 1 Calabah.[38]

A variety of behaviors led to the incarceration of these nondesignated persons. Most were noisy and troublesome at home or in the streets. A woman ran about the streets "naked and shouting"; another woman took off her clothes, shouted loudly, and attacked children; a woman's "silly actions in the streets" caused her hospitalization. A man was sent to the asylum for "causing general confusion in the streets." Another man was "found lying in the middle of the road." A 36-year-old Temne man "entered the general post office and started to throw away books and papers." Some individuals, without provocation, engaged in abusive quarrels with others, threw stones at people or buildings, or attacked persons. A man assaulted "all persons in his house with a knife." Another man "wanted to fight anyone who approached him."

Other persons could not answer questions, or refused to talk, or appeared lost and were unable to care for themselves. One man was declared "non compos mentis"; another man was "found walking in a state of absolute nudity"; and for another individual, the record states: "His behaviour does not seem to be that of a sane individual." A few persons were taken to Kissy for "insane conduct." And often several reasons were given for a patient's hospitalization: one woman, for example, was found "by police creating disturbance in the street"; she had "some grievance against George, the Mendi tribal ruler." She also had "a wild and neglected appearance," and she talked "at random."

While various kinds of conduct might contribute to incarceration, an inmate's discharge was determined largely by the extent to which he or she conformed to a basic pattern of acceptable behavior. Normal appropriate conduct meant being quiet and reserved, eating and sleeping well, and answering questions correctly. A patient was given seven days to settle down, to adjust to hospital life and become agreeable; often the observation period was extended for an additional week or two weeks. The large number of patients who regained composure and were discharged affirms that many clients were able finally to comply with the prevailing norms of behavior.

The speedy return of a patient to the community was also facilitated by the willingness of the patient's family to accept and cope with a mentally ill relative. In addition, a patient's group ties and affiliations, notably ethnic connections, played a role in the discharge process. In numerous instances, particularly when relatives were far away or nonexistent, a tribal ruler or representative in Freetown accepted responsibility for overseeing an ex-mental patient from his tribe. A patient, for example, would be discharged "to the care of the Susu tribal ruler in Freetown." In short, a person was absorbed and sustained by a network of ethnic associations quite distant from that individual's home area.[39]

The fact that many patients entering Kissy Mental Hospital received no psychiatric designation reflected the absence of psychiatric personnel. Sierra Leone did not have a resident psychiatrist; the hospital was administered by African and British general practitioners. The nature of the institution's clientele frustrated the process of psychiatric identification of inmates and, at the same time, illustrated the fundamental character and purpose of the institution. The institution housed the socially deviant, the violent and disruptive, and the homeless, as well as the mentally troubled. Among this clientele - an undifferentiated assortment of inmates - some were clearly mentally ill persons, and others were borderline cases of social deviance and vagrancy. For all, the hospital served as a way station, a depository, a refuge. Therapy remained of minimal concern, but the physical health of inmates was maintained. For a few years, in the mid-1930s, the Kahn test, for detecting syphilis, was routinely administered to incoming patients. Clearly, the chief function of the asylum was providing security and health care to persons viewed as threats, nuisances, or misfits by the wider society. These individuals needed a controlled place and setting that gave them a short period of time to recover and resume acceptable community behavior.

Under these circumstances, the discharge process became a major interest and preoccupation of the hospital administration. The institution was small and understaffed, and it could not accommodate large numbers of patients. If an inmate was not certified insane, or did not pose a danger or embarrassment to others, that individual had to be discharged - to friends or relatives, to a tribal representative, to a hospital or infirmary, to prison, or, increasingly, in the late 1930s, to the King George VI Memorial Home.

THE PERSISTENCE OF THE POOR

Most of the persons in the nondesignated group were poor, a socioeconomic status common to mental patients in all psychiatric categories. Poverty remained the most basic and enduring characteristic of the mad, bad, and deviant housed at Kissy Mental Hospital. Some were cases of abject destitution, a condition that carried a unique status and stigma. Not only was the destitute individual very poor, clinging to the bottom stratum of the social order, that person was also an outsider, someone without social ties or relationships. Other poor people received support from friends, a family, a tribal association, or some religious or community group. The destitute individual was devoid of normal connections, had no possibility of acquiring them, and became further isolated when incapacitated.

Identified as a "destitute," a "pauper," or a "vagrant," this type of patient was transferred, usually after a few days or weeks in the asylum, to an infirmary or the memorial home. A destitute beggar, for example, suffering from Parkinson's disease, spent only one day in the mental hospital before he was sent to another institution. After three months at Kissy, another man, who was admitted without any belongings, went to the memorial home. Many of the destitute cases were elderly persons, arriving in a weak physical condition. On admission, for instance, a 52-year-old Mende man was "restless and weak," "dehydrated," and "markedly emaciated"; he also showed "elephantiasis of the scrotum," as well as hemorrhoids. He remained "confused and noisy" and died four days after arriving.[40]

Along with the destitute, many of the insane poor at the mental hospital were unskilled laborers and farmers. Throughout the colonial period, this segment of the poor remained on a treadmill of economic stagnation and deprivation. Their circumstances embraced casual and infrequent work, low wages, which always lagged behind prices and inflation, and indebtedness. During World War II, 80 percent of the workers of Freetown were indebted.

Petty traders, chiefly female, also made up a sizeable number of the insane poor. Sierra Leone women were part of the tradition of female marketing in West Africa. Some 85 to 95 percent of traders were women engaged in the streets selling such items as cooked food or baked goods, fruit, and cigarettes, in small quantities to supply the poor. At Kissy Mental Hospital, traders formed the largest group of female patients among those who specified an occupation. The other most frequently listed occupations for female inmates included seamstress, laundress, housewife, and to a lesser extent, hawker, cook, and servant.

Young people in the crafts or trades constituted another layer of the urban poor. Such individuals had only primary schooling, and their best hope for survival was apprenticeship in a trade. Throughout West Africa, most apprentices were males under 25 years of age, and they spent three to five years acquiring whatever skills they could pick up. They went unpaid, receiving a daily meal, and, over a period of time, a few presents. While this was an exploitative arrangement that held down wages, it did provide inexpensive training, sustained the crafts, and allowed overcrowded trades such as tailoring, as well as decaying ones such as blacksmithing and leatherwork, to endure. The major trades represented by mental patients at the Kissy asylum included carpenter, tailor, stonemason, goldsmith, blacksmith, and shoemaker. Some of the male inmates also were fishermen or seamen, two traditionally low-paying occupations.

Young male immigrants, particularly the Kroo from Liberia and the escaped slaves or freedmen from Yorubaland, represented another segment of the Freetown poor. Living in clusters of shacks in the poorer areas of the community, they took jobs others refused, notably heavy manual labor, earned little, and brawled frequently. They were a dominant group in prison and in the mental asylum. For certain other elements of the poor, crime was a source of income. Much of it involved offenses against property. Most of the individuals were poor - the unemployed and those without a trade - and often they stole simply to eat. As noted earlier, criminals subject to erratic behavior, especially violent conduct, and prisoners from the jail, who seemed mentally troubled and boisterous, were committed to the Kissy hospital.[41]

A PROFILE

In sum, the patients at the mental hospital reflected the social realities of a society in which the masses of people never received a regular wage. They represented the poor - a broad amorphous class formed around a matrix of interrelationships, roles, identifications, and occupations, ranging from the destitute to the casual laborer, the petty trader, the immigrant worker, and the criminal. Poverty was the social basis, and a fundamental fact, of colonial life.

Other demographic patterns emerge to broaden this profile of the colonial insane. Over these years from 1905 to 1959, the ethnic groups with the largest percentage of patients at the mental hospital were the Mende, Temne, and Krio, a pattern apparent in almost every psychiatric category. The Mende and Temne were the largest ethnic units of Sierra Leone; this numerical superiority was reflected in the higher number of mental patients.

Krios formed a small percentage of the total population but were numerous in Freetown and the western part of the country, the area close to the mental hospital. The significant influx of Krios to the Kissy institution conforms to a basic trend of public utilization of mental health services throughout the world: propinquity to a mental hospital facilitates and encourages local acceptance of the institution, as well as admission of those nearby residents who require care and incarceration. Krio familiarity with Western values and institutions also facilitated use and acceptance of the asylum.

Other ethnic groups with representation in the hospital included Kroo, Sherbro, Susu, and Limba. Foreign ethnics, residing in Freetown for generations, notably Foulah, Jollof, and Mandingo, formed a percentage of Kissy patients. Only a few inmates came from tribes located in the more remote eastern areas of the country.

In terms of age and gender, across most psychiatric designations, young men and middle-aged women seemed the most prone to mental disturbance. While men and women of all ages were evident, men in their twenties and early thirties and women in their thirties and forties, the period of middle age for twentieth century Africa, formed the major group of Kissy patients. And a most striking related fact was the overwhelming prevalence of males to females. For every kind of illness, there were more males than females; in most instances, the males were three times the number of females. Madness in colonial Sierra Leone was clearly a predominantly male disorder.

NOTES

1. This chapter is based largely on an analysis of the case records of patients who were admitted to Kissy Mental Hospital between 1905 and 1959. These consist of voluminous histories of clients, bound into large, oversize books. The information kept on each patient includes gender, age, dates of admission and discharge or death, tribe or ethnic identity, religion, occupation, and psychiatric designation. In many instances, the information is incomplete. For example, a patient's religion was rarely recorded after 1916. The records are most consistent regarding gender and dates of arrival and departure.

A standard pattern of entering information determined the narrative of the course of institutional life of each inmate. Usually the reasons for incarceration were given, and for the patient's first week, daily notes were made. Monthly remarks were recorded for the first six months, and thereafter half yearly notations were maintained. The exception to this pattern occurred when a patient became ill and was under special treatment.

2. T. A. Lambo, "Neuro-psychiatric Syndromes Associated with Human Trypanosomiasis in Tropical Africa," *Acta Psychiatrica Scandinavica* 42 (1966): 474-84; M. J. Field, "Chronic Psychosis in Rural Ghana," *British Journal of Psychiatry* 114 (1968): 31-33.

3. National Archives of Sierra Leone, cited as SLA, Case Records (hereafter CR) numbers 123, 129, 135, 202, 238 (1905-16); 689 (1919-22); 984 (1925-28); 4638 (1938-43); 4995 (1947-51).

4. SLA, CR numbers 173, 180, 208, 224 (1905-16); 814, 815, 823, 844 (1922-25).

5. SLA, CR numbers 226, 264, 267, 273, 303, 454, 462, 485 (1905-16); 555 (1916-19); 668, 673, 678, 759, 761, 765 (1919-22); 824 (1922-25); 1070, 2054 (1925-28); 2070, 3073, 3087, 3089, 3099 (1928-31); 4096 (1943-45); 4805, 4883 (1945-47); 4936, 5005, 5049, 5133 (1947-51); 5366, 5372, 5373,

5450, 5453, 5456, 5465, 5487, 5488, 5497, 5512, 5524, 5548, 5550, 5555, 5565, 5601 (1954-59).

6. SLA, CR numbers 145, 161, 197, 248, 262, 274, 277, 296, 307, 311, 323, 339, 343, 357, 360, 376, 386, 396, 419, 446, 466, 469, 489, 491 (1905-16); 514, 518, 552, 568, 575, 621 (1916-19); 677, 763, 790 (1919-22); 900, 923, 937, 966, 967 (1922-25); 1020, 1049, 2031 (1925-28); 2090, 2092, 2097, 3003, 3063, 3075 (1928-31); 4106, 4130, 4171 (1931-34); 4399, 4439 (1934-38); 4479, 4480, 4514, 4543, 4546, 4556, 4596, 4598, 4608, 4609, 4623 (1938-43); 4800, 4807, 4839, 4879, 4889 (1945-47); 4993, 5079 (1947-51); 5403, 5411, 5449, 5517, 5531, 5532, 5545, 5582 (1954-59).

7. SLA, CR number 234 (1905-16).

8. SLA, CR numbers 735 (1925-28); 2064, 3021 (1928-31); 4364 (1931-34); 4802 (1945-47); 4925, 4933, 4957, 5024 (1947-51); 5382, 5432, 5463, 5576 (1954-59).

9. SLA, CR numbers 735 (1919-22); 929 (1922-25); 1011 (1925-28); 4550, 4557, 4626, 4646 (1938-43); 4698 (1943-45); 4920, 4988, 4996, 5022, 5095, 5102, 5104, 5135 (1947-51).

10. SLA, CR number 735 (1919-22).

11. SLA, CR numbers 181, 201, 206, 218, 245, 255, 257, 261, 268, 299, 310, 331, 334, 348, 359, 362, 363, 383, 394, 429, 447, 471, 505 (1905-16); 521, 546, 584, 606, 628, 637 (1916-19); 672, 697, 723, 724, 732, 788, 789, 800 (1919-22); 849, 851, 853, 878, 882, 884, 889, 918, 933, 950, 960, 963 (1922-25); 981, 991, 1023, 1065, 2016, 2027, 2037 (1922-25); 4045, 4052 (1931-34); 4295 (1934-38); 4457 (1938-43); 4671 (1943-45); 5386, 5427 (1954-59).

12. SLA, CR numbers 121, 132, 143, 154, 164, 183, 191, 195, 198, 223, 226, 227, 228, 242, 249, 297, 304, 315, 319, 324, 329, 349, 411, 421, 445, 451, 465, 470, 474 (1905-16); 566, 602, 638 (1916-19); 701, 715, 748 (1919-22); 813, 836, 839, 859, 870, 888, 899, 906, 908, 914, 922, 935, 954 (1922-25); 2012 (1925-28); 3007, 3052, 3055, 3086 (1928-31); 4072 (1931-34); 4588, 4597 (1938-43); 4705 (1943-45); 4929, 4999 (1947-51); 5365, 5372, 5374, 5375, 5479, 5565, 5571, 5577, 5578, 5589 (1954-59).

13. Charles R. Swift and Tolani Asuni, *Mental Health and Disease in Africa: With Special Reference to Africa South of the Sahara* (Edinburgh: Churchill Livingstone, 1975), 183-85.

14. SLA, CR numbers 158, 185, 192, 199, 200, 233, 234, 237, 332, 387, 407, 416, 476, 506 (1905-16); 675, 680, 740, 770, 773 (1919-22); 904, 939, 957, 962 (1922-25); 1045, 1085, 2045 (1925-28); 2067, 3005, 3020, 3081 (1928-31): 4004, 4008, 4086, 4094, 4102, 4150, 4151, 4177 (1931-34); 4282 (1934-38);

4568, 4618, 4659 (1938-43); 4684, 4687, 4694, 4711, 4718, 4778 (1943-45); 4799, 4809, 4874 (1945-47); 5020, 5050, 5060, 5090, 5136 (1947-51); 5376, 5379, 5449 (1954-59).

15. Cases designated acute mania in SLA, CR 1905-16; 1916-19; 1919-22; 1922-25; 1925-28; 1928-31; 1931-34; 1934-38; 1938-43; 1943-45; 1945-47; 1947-51; 1954-59.

16. SLA, CR numbers 211, 214, 215, 225, 235, 236, 282, 283, 285, 301, 302, 308, 312, 316, 322, 344, 345, 353, 356, 358, 361, 366, 370, 380, 385, 393, 405, 477, 492 (1905-16); 546, 550, 586, 594, 647 (1916-19); 2014 (1925-28); 4463 (1938-43); 4982, 5983 (1947-51).

17. SLA, CR numbers 122, 126, 131, 144, 149, 150, 158, 177, 188 (1905-16); 528, 556 (1916-19); 809 (1922-25).

18. SLA, CR numbers 172, 174, 179 (1905-16).

19. SLA, CR number 5520 (1943-59).

20. SLA, CR numbers 4743 (1943-45); 4895 (1945-47); 5462, 5572 (1954-59).

21. SLA, CR number 457 (1905-16).

22. SLA, CR number 4020 (1928-31).

23. SLA, CR number 676 (1905-16).

24. SLA, CR number 897 (1922-25).

25. SLA, CR numbers 4671, 4672 (1943-45); 5089, 5140 (1947-51).

26. SLA, CR number 675 (1919-22).

27. SLA, CR numbers 402, 404, 507 (1905-16); 850, 856, 883, 866, 895, 899 (1922-25); 4146 (1931-34); 4276 (1934-38).

28. SLA, CR number 504 (1905-16); 805 (1919-22); 819, 893, 894 (1922-25); 5058, 5060, 5073, 5100 (1947-51).

29. SLA, CR numbers 2011 (1925-28); 3044 (1928-31).

30. SLA, CR numbers 5030, 5036, 5037, 5039, 5040, 5042, 5044, 5052, 5054, 5055, 5056, 5083, 5109 (1947-51).

31. SLA, CR numbers 2036 (1925-28); 5136, 5148 (1947-51).

32. SLA, CR numbers 3078 (1928-31); 4581, 4603 (1938-43); 4714, 4757, 4761 (1943-45); 4847, 4849, 4862, 4885, 4887 (1945-47); 4963, 4967, 4971, 5004, 5068, 5092, 5094, 5137 (1947-51); 5380, 5384, 5395, 5396, 5405, 5414, 5521, 5423, 5424, 5428, 5436, 5447, 5455, 5466, 5478, 5480, 5481, 5492, 5504, 5508, 5525, 5527, 5541, 5543, 5556, 5560, 5563, 5591, 5592 (1954-59).

33. SLA, CR numbers 531 (1916-19); 837, 840, 843, 848, 857, 860, 867, 874, 881, 885, 972, 978 (1922-25); 1014, 1095 (1925-28); 3043, 4019 (1928-31); 4062 (1931-34); 4423 (1934-38); 4657, 4737 (1938-43); 4846 (1945-47); 5028, 5046, 5057, 5067, 5071, 5076, 5081, 5084, 5095, 5097, 5099, 5104, 5110,

5114, 5120, 5121, 5132, 5134, 5138, 5141, 5142 (1947-51).

34. SLA, CR numbers 141, 202, 211, 238, 262, 357, 378, 408, 414, 432 (1905-16); 550 (1916-19); 820, 837, 838 (1922-25); 1046, 2018, 2043 (1925-28); 3030, 3070, 3097 (1928-31); 4075 (1931-34); 4237,4259, 4348, 4396, 4406, 4410, 4417, 4426, 4431 (1934-38); 4442, 4443, 4461, 4475, 4490, 4494, 4501, 4513, 4535, 4540, 4583, 4594, 4603, 4625, 4640 (1938-43); 4675, 4678, 4680, 4686, 4699, 4708, 4713, 4714, 4715 (1943-45); 4783, 4802, 4836, 4839, 4847, 4849, 4851, 4864, 4866, 4867, 4869, 4878, 4880, 4892, 4896, 4906, 4911, 4912 (1945-47); 4921, 4935, 4952, 4961, 4962, 4963, 4976, 4987, 5010, 5022, 5024, 5041, 5044, 5056, 5087, 5113 (1947-51); 5397, 5319, 5324, 5325, 5429, 5430, 5543, 5544, 5552, 5563, 5574, 5593 (1954-59).

An excellent discussion of cross-cultural delusions is John C. Burnham, "Psychotic Delusions as a Key to Historical Cultures: Tasmania, 1830-1940," *Journal of Social History* 13 (1980): 368-83.

35. SLA, CR numbers 313 (1905-16); 776, 802 (1919-22).

36. SLA, CR numbers 388, 407, 410, 413, 424 (1905-16); 554, 585, 600 (1916-19); 780, 948 (1922-25); 982 (1925-28); 3028 (1928-31); 4083, 4183 (1931-34); 4369, 4389, 4432 (1934-38); 4456, 4492, 4512, 4531, 4536, 4556, 4647, 4657 (1938-43); 4706, 4716, 4721 (1943-45); 4822, 4829, 4835, 4861, 4913 (1945-47); 4917, 4959, 4960 (1947-51); 5069, 5111, 5444, 5445, 5598 (1954-59).

37. SLA, CR mumbers 126, 137, 189, 228, 230, 233, 234, 253, 260, 262, 271, 304, 316, 324, 326, 337, 338, 368, 408, 420, 436, 441, 450, 456 (1905-16); 513, 564, 637 (1916-19); 705, 716, 744, 751, 771, 772, 779 (1919-22); 822, 827, 934, 981 (1922-25); js (no number), 986, 1000, 2048, 2058, 2060 (1925-28); 3012, 3016, 3018, 4001 (1928-31); 4006, 4039, 4041, 4074, 4077, 4130, 4132, 4146, 4136, 4173 (1931-34); 4257, 4285, 4293, 4408, 4416 (1934-38); 4469, 4483, 4489, 4504, 4524, 4540, 4657, 4658, 4664 (1938-43); 4699, 4734 (1943-45); 4799, 4803, 4811, 4814, 4818, 4821, 4840, 4850, 4854, 4859, 4864, 4872, 4877, 4881, 4884, 4887, 4889, 4895 (1945-47); 4939, 4945, 4955, 4957, 4967, 4988, 5000, 5006, 5013, 5014, 5020, 5022, 5032, 5039, 5040, 5046, 5053, 5065, 5074, 5076, 5084, 5094, 5114, 5121, 5127, 5141, 5149 (1947-51); 5377, 5388, 5395, 5396, 5401, 5403, 5414, 5416, 5420, 5429,5434, 5449, 5457, 5474, 5474, 5486, 5487, 5490, 5499, 5502, 5503, 5504, 5509, 5537, 5582, 5598, 5610 (1954-59).

38. Nondesignated cases in SLA, CR (1905-16); (1916-19); (1919-22); (1922-25); (1925-28); (1928-31); (1931-34); (1934-

38); (1938-43); (1943-45); (1945-47); (1947-51); (1954-59).

39. For the development of ethnic communities in Freetown, see Barbara E. Harrell-Bond, Allen M. Howard, and David E. Skinner, *Community Leadership and the Transformation of Freetown, 1801-1976* (The Hague: Mouton Publishers, 1978); and Michael Banton, *West African City: A Study of Tribal Life in Freetown* (London: Oxford University Press, 1957).

40. Examples of destitute cases include CR numbers 2091 (1928-31); 4362, 4371 (1934-38); 4805, 4833, 4837, 4859 (1945-47); 4984 (1947-51); 5380 (1955-59).

41. John Iliffe, *The African Poor: A History* (London: Cambridge University Press, 1987), 172, 174-75, 182. This is an excellent study of African poverty.

5 Change and Continuity

In the years after Sierra Leone became an independent nation, the types of patients entering Kissy Mental Hospital came to differ significantly from those of the colonial past. Many of the changes were manifestations of the new social problems affecting a developing nation in the closing decades of the twentieth century. The major indicators of social maladjustment, notably crime, family disruptions, and drug and alcohol addiction, showed increasingly higher rates of frequency and volume. Such difficult problems were exacerbated by a society trapped in economic malaise. The patients admitted to Kissy hospital reflected these new and fluctuating social stresses. In growing numbers, the facility accepted persons overwhelmed by marital troubles, alcoholism, and drug dependency; many presented a record of criminal activities and general psychopathology. Psychiatric nomenclatures and illnesses evolved. Clients suffered, particularly, for example, from the mental disorders, schizophrenia and depression, which were, worldwide, the two most prominent diagnoses of psychotic diseases of the late twentieth century.

As in the past, however, numerous patients were labeled with the various kinds of mania, as well as GPI, epilepsy, and mental retardation. Also as in the earlier period, cases of parasuicide, witchcraft, and religious and other delusional states were well represented. In addition, the persistence of large numbers of unclassified patients remained a continuing phenomenon. Transient psychosis was now the term applied to many of the nondesignated cases. It was used to identify this short-lived condition, characterized frequently by aggressive outbursts, followed by periods of confusion, with the person returning to normalcy within a few weeks or months. A relatively brief hospital stay was typical for patients incapacitated by other kinds of psychiatric disorders.

The basic demographics of age, with the young more represented than the old, and ethnic makeup, with the major groups persisting, remained consistent with the past. And a most obvious fact prevailed: young men, often exhibiting disruptive and threatening behavior, dominated the admissions to Kissy hospital.[1]

PSYCHOPATHIC PERSONALITY

Psychopathic personality was a new psychiatric designation utilized in postcolonial Sierra Leone. Between 1960 and the 1980s, a group of nineteen patients - seventeen men and two women - consisting largely of prisoners and the unemployed, were placed in this category. Their lengths of hospitalization ranged from three days to nine years. A few absconded; several were criminals and were returned to prison after a period of observation at Kissy. Some were cases of alcohol and drug dependency and had several readmissions. These psychopathic persons were often characterized as "utterly amoral," unrepentant, and violent. In some instances, they had committed a heinous crime. A man, incarcerated in prison for killing an 8-year-old child, was observed in the hospital for two months; one of the women was charged with murdering a child, albeit she denied and remained indifferent to that fact. Four young, unemployed men, teenage dropouts, engaged in random and uncontrollable violence.

Other types of compulsive activity characterized the behavior of some psychopaths, namely obsessive thievery, alcohol and drug addiction, and persistent, ungovernable sexual actions. The intolerable behavior of psychopathic thieves was often exacerbated by the very act of being caught stealing. Invariably, with the alcohol and drug cases, the men lost jobs and got into fights.

Persons guilty of sexual abuse took a defensive posture, blaming their victims for criminal action. A man, for instance, charged with assaulting a 9-year-old girl, accused the child of sexually abusing him. Another case of sexual dysfunction was an exhibitionist, a single middle-aged man sent to prison for disorderly conduct and indecent exposure. In most respects, he was a typical representative of this group of psychopaths: isolated, alienated, disoriented, and compulsive, he had no family or friends. Living on the fringe of society, he was absorbed in his obsession.

DOMESTIC STRESSES

Beginning after World War II, domestic problems, notably marital troubles, figured prominently among the factors mentioned in referrals of mentally distressed persons to Kissy Mental Hospital. This was a new development, a new pattern that reflected the changing nature of the institution's clientele. In the colonial period, single men formed the majority of patients in every psychiatric category as well as in the nondesignated sector. After 1945, during the late colonial era, and becoming more obvious in the years between 1960 and the 1980s, single men remained a large element in the pool of mental patients, but increasingly, married individuals, both male and female, madeup a significantly large group of inmates. And family situations, particularly turbulent relationships between the sexes, had often become a contributing reason for incarceration.

Between 1945 and the 1980s, 130 patients, sixty-eight female and sixty-two male, complained about anxieties caused by domestic strife. Among the women, there were six instances of worry over financial matters. A 24-year-old Krio woman of nondesignated status became mentally distressed when child support payments, regularly received for a year, abruptly ended. Another nondesignated Krio housewife, "a heavy drinker," was disturbed that her husband was not maintaining her and her children. A 34-year-old Mandingo woman quarrelled with her husband because he did not provide for "her financial needs." An old Temne woman, a case of senile dementia, was reduced to begging when deserted by her husband and son. Two single woman were distraught after being abandoned by their boyfriends: a 19-year-old pregnant woman, who turned to alcohol for relief, lamented over the irresponsibility of her boyfriend; a 27-year-old Muslim nurse was despondent over her suitor who had left for America and was not sending money to support their two children. Restless and agitated, she believed that "people were talking about her."

Victims and perpetrators of domestic violence were sent to Kissy. Beaten wives found a refuge. A woman sustaining head injuries inflicted by her husband was maintained for six months at the hospital. After a severe beating, a 40-year-old Foulah woman left her husband and resided at the asylum for two months. A 32-

year-old Sierra Leonean housewife, married for twelve years, said she loved her husband for nine of those years, but then violent quarrels began, during which he frequently slapped her. Following a noisy and difficult wrangle, the police intervened. She was taken to the mental hospital, where she remained for two weeks before being discharged to the care of her mother.

A tragic and brutal case involved a 45-year-old Mende man who discovered that his wife had been unfaithful to him. He beat her to death, was designated a criminal lunatic, and kept in the mental institution until he died, fourteen years later. Another instance of extreme violence was a 19-year-old Mende student who raped his girlfriend because she would not marry him. A 50-year-old man, married for fourteen years, started beating his wife for no apparent reason. While she grew despondent, not so much because of the beatings but over his foolish practice of giving money away, he was placed in the mental hospital. A middle-aged Temne man, who severely beat his wife during a quarrel, was isolated in the asylum for eleven months, at which point he absconded.

A few jealous husbands vented their anger and inflicted violence on the lovers of their wives. A houseboy had an affair with one man's wife; a neighbor loved another man's spouse. In each case, after fighting the lover, the husband was taken to Kissy hospital for observation, declared sane, and, in time, sent to prison on a charge of disorderly conduct. Some husbands became mentally unhinged and violent when deserted by their wives. For example, after a Krio man learned that his wife in England wanted a divorce, he exhibited disorderly behavior, attacking and insulting people. Over a year later, he accepted a divorce arrangement and was discharged, on parole, from the hospital.

Various kinds of violent actions led some wives to leave their spouses. A wife, along with her two children, refused to live with a husband who jumped on people and upset carts in the marketplace. The two wives of a farmer left him because of his erratic and threatening behavior: he chased relatives with a knife and tried to kill one of his father's wives. In another case, violent quarreling among the father's wives led the son's only wife to leave the household.

Violent disputes among relatives brought clients to Kissy. A 52-year-old married man, suffering from schizophrenia, fought physically with in-laws; another man displayed continuous aggression toward his parents; and other patients related to family members in turbulent and threatening ways. Once such individuals were placed in the mental hospital, the family frequently was relieved and expected that the disturbed relative would remain institutionalized for a long time. A 19-year-old Susu man, designated as a schizophrenia paranoid type, who at home ran after relatives with a knife, remained at Kissy for twenty-one years. A middle-aged Sierra Leonean woman stayed in the asylum for over a decade; relatives insisted on her continued incarceration. The family of a 26-year-old Limba man refused responsibility for him. Excitable and incoherent, he attacked others and destroyed their clothing; he was kept in the hospital for three years. The relatives of a 29-year-old Temne woman, who was "uncontrollable at home," wanted her in the hospital. She remained at the facility for eight months, a relatively short time. This case, however, typified others in which families admitted an unwillingness to look after or tolerate violently disposed relatives, and in which the hospitalization of the disturbed person for only a brief period brought some relief to a situation of stress and strain.

Some wives complained about the indifference, emotional aridity, or hostility of their husbands. A 28-year-old Krio woman, suffering from manic depressive psychosis, charged that her husband did not "treat her well," and that he showed no concern when she threatened suicide. His pervasive detachment, the wife asserted, made her depressed and withdrawn, causing her repeated relapses and hospital admissions.

While depression overcome some women of indifferent husbands, other wives retaliated, demanding retribution from spouses who had rebuffed them. A Temne housewife, laboring with schizophrenia, assaulted her husband with a machete, claiming that he "did not care for her." A 38-year-old woman with two children became violent at home and in the streets, asserting a desire to mutilate her husband. Married for four years, she was initially happy with the union. Her husband, however, gave her no affection; she grew annoyed and excited, and began displaying "abnormal behavior."

There were a few cases of rejection, followed by total abandonment, a situation leaving considerable emotional pain. A woman, for example, became withdrawn and "very uncommunicative" when deserted by her Gambian boyfriend, who had promised to marry her and had fathered three of her children. When the husband of a 50-year-old housewife deserted her, the woman sank into a state of general depression that lasted several years. The disappearance of a boyfriend of a young woman left her so tense and anxious that she was hospitalized for eight weeks; after discharge, she spent months trying to find him. A 30-year-old housewife was anxious and dejected after she learned that her husband discovered her affair with another man. Upset that he might leave her, she ran through the streets, stopping and asking people to intervene on her behalf, pleading with them to ask forgiveness from her husband. Soon after the marriage of a 38-year-old Krio schoolteacher ended in separation, the man became lonely and unhappy. He worried and lost weight and, eventually, spent three months in the mental hospital. He absorbed himself in religious devotions and services and tried several times to win back his wife.

Two difficult and emotionally tense marital problems affected the female clients more than the males: a childless marriage and the jealous relationships engendered within a polygamous marriage. Some wives were clearly preoccupied with their inability to have children. This matter became especially stressful when the husband rejected and left an infertile wife for another woman. For example, a 46-year-old Krio housewife, married and childless for seventeen years, suspicious about her spouse's fidelity, discovered that her husband had acquired a girlfriend who bore him a child. Upset and restless, she experienced bouts of weeping and severe depression. In another case, a Mende woman was overcome with suicidal visions soon after her husband announced he was leaving her because she was childless. She dreamed of being sold as a witch and told to cut her throat with a knife. She heard voices announcing her death. For over a year, she was in a state of depression at the mental hospital.

A 51-year-old Krio woman also heard voices; she had a child out of wedlock, but during fifteen years of marriage she remained barren. She stated that upon hearing her husband's voice ordering her out of the house, she went into the streets. She spent three and a half years at the Kissy hospital. While these women brooded over their conditions, the cause of infertility was a moot question. One woman, institutionalized for eighteen years, attributed her childlessness to her mother's witchcraft and sister's destruction of "all her eggs." Sorcery, the machinations of some evil force, was a popular and acceptable way of explaining female, and male, sterility.

Polygamy, a basic part of traditional society, has remained widespread throughout Sierra Leone and all of Africa. By the mid-twentieth century, under the impact of urbanization, and the emergence of a more fluid social and economic order, as well as Christian and Western influences, monogamy gained social support, particularly among the educated. Challenges to tradition created conflict and a confusion of roles; the unexpected appearance of a new spouse or spouses produced awkward relationships within polygamous marriages. This kind of situation caused stress and anxiety and led to the mental disturbance of several female patients sent to Kissy.

A Mende woman, for example, was happily married until her husband took several other wives. At that point, frequent quarrels and violent scenes ensued. She moved out and stayed with friends, but she became morose and dejected and was sent to the mental hospital, where she remained for seventeen years. Another woman, in a polygamous union of eight, took physical abuse from her husband. Subject to fits of weeping and depression, she spent six months at Kissy and was discharged to the care of her daughter. In two other cases, middle-aged women with children grew distraught and jealous when their husbands brought home new wives. And one of the wives of a dual marriage appeared to worry herself into severe depression, believing that her husband was more interested in the other wife.

Aside from these women torn by the frustrations of polygamous marriages, some female patients experienced intense emotional pain over the sudden discovery of an unfaithful husband or boyfriend. An ex-mental patient, returning home from the hospital, learned that her husband had a girlfriend. The shock of this disclosure, coupled with the rudeness of the girlfriend, contributed to the wife's relapse and return to the mental hospital. One vexatious case dealt with a 28-year-old woman who had married and had two children in another country. Her husband left her for another woman, and she returned to Sierra Leone without her children. Upset, deluded, and disruptive, she was kept in the Kissy hospital for three months. A few women, surprised and overcome by their spouses' involvements with other women, attempted to find refuge in alcohol and became problem drinkers.

Sickness and death generated emotional crises in both husbands and wives. In some cases, mental disorder severed a relationship. A Mende trader, burdened by GPI, had six wives: two died and the remaining four, unwilling to tolerate his mental condition, deserted him. After a year in the hospital, he was discharged to the care of his son. A few husbands were also intolerant of a spouse's sickness, abandoning a mentally deranged or physically sick wife.

Deaths affected women more profoundly than men. Of fifteen cases dealing with the deaths of a spouse or a close relative or a child, only two male clients were involved. In each instance, the wife of a middle-aged man had died, leaving the husband emotionally stunned and apathetic. Both men did recover quickly and return to a normal life. The most emotionally devastated women were those who experienced multiple family deaths. After losing her father, husband, and son, a Krio housewife, diagnosed as suffering from depression, wanted to die and attempted suicide, cutting her throat. She was in the hospital for a year and a half. Another middle-aged woman confessed that she had no interest in living; her husband and nine of her ten children had died. A 45-year-old housewife also felt a profound indifference to life; she had lost all contacts with her eight children, and her husband had recently passed away.

For a few women, just a husband's death precipitated mental disorder. One woman, a 30-year-old Limba trader, attributed her own violent behavior to the demise of her spouse. And many of the women patients were distressed over the death of a son or a daughter. In all these cases, the time of recovery extended over several months. One long-term patient is recorded: a 51-year-old Sierra Leonean who became violent and irrational when her daughter died. She was maintained at the hospital for seventeen years.

People who were overwrought and caught in other types of stressful domestic situations were sent to Kissy. A Temne woman, estranged from her spouse, worried that her husband would take away her 2-year-old child. Earlier, the police had intervened when he forcibly abducted the infant. Another separated woman had lost custody of her son and was confronted daily with hostile relatives. She broke down and engaged in destructive behavior; occasionally, she saw "a black devil." A 12-year-old schoolboy, designated a schizophrenic, disturbed by a turbulent household in which many children quarreled continuously, took drugs and claimed that a "devil was commanding him to kill."

Two students, failing university exams, disrupted familial tranquillity. Unable to pass a qualifying exam for entrance to law school, one was told to leave a British university. He returned to Sierra Leone, underwent native treatment, and was incarcerated at the asylum. The other student failed a final exam at Fourah Bay College. He turned down an opportunity to retake the exam, refusing to study or work. His repeated outbursts of aggression led to his removal, on several occasions, to the Kissy hospital.

The detrimental effect of a divorce on a son was evident in a case of a 24-year-old clerk classified as an unstable personality.

When his parents' marriage ended and they separated, he was unable to relate to either his father or mother. He became abusive to elders, neglected his appearance, and started drinking alcoholic beverages. After repeated exhibitions of antisocial behavior, he experienced relapses and readmissions to the mental hospital.

Two men entertained suicide as a way out of a painful domestic problem: a husband, fed up with a nagging wife, wanted to end his life; a 20-year-old Sierra Leonean attempted to drown himself after fighting with his mother over his girlfriend.

A similar domestic setting in another case produced a different result. The mother did not like her son's girlfriend, who resided in the home. She was convinced that the girlfriend was "planning evil things to kill her." Distraught by this fear, she took to drinking, ran about half-naked, and abused people.

Homesickness contributed to the mental breakdown of a 46-year-old married Temne man. He left his family to take a job far away as a road laborer. While his work was good, he became lonely and returned often to his native village, disregarding his job. For this negligence, he eventually was sacked. Back home, confused and agitated, he deteriorated mentally, and, at times, would terrify the household. The family, after unsuccessful native treatments, sent him to Kissy, where he remained for five years.

Some male patients had faced stresses on the job as well as the disruptions of a failing marriage. A Krio schoolteacher, who wanted a divorce, confessed that "teaching was a strain," and said the headmaster was "not sympathetic" to his problems. A police constable, a Mende man separated from his wife, worried that he was not "satisfying his boss." And a Limba railroad worker, whose wife had left him for another man, believed that coworkers were talking about him.

A demographic overview of the 130 patients anxious about or tormented by domestic troubles reveals that the majority were short-term inmates with a nondesignated psychiatric status. Among those diagnosed depressive, women predominated; men were more numerous in the groupings of schizophrenics. The ethnic makeup of these patients was largely Krio, Mende, and Temne; this representation corresponded to the largest ethnic groups in the Freetown area. A large proportion of the women identified themselves as housewives; the men came from an assortment of trades and menial occupations. The majority of the men were under the age of 30; most of the women were over 30. This finding confirms a basic pattern found in other psychiatric categories, suggesting that young men and middle-aged women were the most likely to be institutionalized for mental disturbance.

ALCOHOLISM AND DRUG ADDICTION

After World War II, drug and alcohol abuse became a common reason given in admission notes for the incarceration of clients at Kissy Mental Hospital. Throughout the country, the most popular alcoholic beverage was omole, a local moonshine whiskey. The most abused drug still was diamba, better known as *Cannabis sativa* or marijuana. Palm wine, beer, and gin were consumed by heavy drinkers; some drug users took amphetamines and a substance called "datura stramonium," known locally as "kube jarra," a term meaning "it cures everything." The hard drugs, namely cocaine, heroin, and morphine, were not widely used in Sierra Leone. These drugs were observed largely in cases involving foreigners who smuggled narcotics into the country for their own personal use.

Between 1945 and the early 1980s, there were 242 admissions related to some kind of chemical dependence - 199 men and 43 women. Of these clients, only a few women took drugs; most of them, over 95 percent, were problem drinkers. The men, on the other hand, indulged in drugs as well as alcohol, and in many instances, they were both alcoholics and drug addicts. Young, single men formed the largest element of drug abusers: many were teenagers, most were below the age of 30. Women alcoholics ranged from 18 to 62, and the majority were married and over 25 years of age.

The elderly, both male and female, constituted a very small part of this group of alcohol and drug users. Two cases typified the older addict: one man, designated an alcoholic, had been "drinking all his life - 30 years," and was now "demented and troublesome." Physically weak and uncoordinated, he shook when he walked. After a year in the mental hospital, he was transferred to the memorial home. Another man, a beggar, spent several short terms in prison. He would bite and throw stones at people and was admitted and discharged from Kissy hospital a few times. He too was sent to the memorial home. In both of these cases, the older dependent occupied a fringe status in the community, alienated and removed from family, relatives, and friends.

A striking feature of the addict population was the large number of students and unemployed people - a corollary, in effect, to the predominance of young persons in the group. There were also prisoners, sailors, farmers, and laborers, as well as housewives. The most prominent ethnic groups were Krio, Mende, and Temne.

There were a few cases of persons involved in only an infrequent drinking or drug episode. One night after work, for example, a 23-year-old Kissi driver drank too much wine and fell ill. He went to the hospital in Freetown, became violent, and was sent to Kissy. A week later he was discharged, sane and rational. This was an atypical case. Most of the alcohol and drug clients were seriously ill from longstanding abuse and dependency. Many were identified as suffering from alcoholism, alcoholic dementia, or alcoholic psychosis. Some were diagnosed as being in a "diamba confusional state," an "omole confusional state," or a "toxic confusional state." Also, in the case notes of some patients, an informal reference clarified the client's troubles. A middle-aged Mende woman, for instance, had "a long history of drinking palm wine"; another woman had been "drinking illicit gin for years"; a Loko man had a "history of heavy drinking of locally distilled spirits." Several patients had repeated admissions and were recorded simply as "a problem drinker," "a known alcoholic," "a chronic alcoholic," "a known drug addict," or "a diamba addict."

Most of these patients remained in the institution for a short period. The length of stay of a typical substance abuse resident was two months; some inmates were readmitted several times. They suffered from the long-term effects of alcoholism and were often recorded as experiencing delirium tremens. The largest number of alcohol and drug clients were incarcerated for threatening or committing an act of violence. A diamba addict, for example, a prisoner from the Gold Coast, attacked people with a machete; another man, who indulged in "excessive drinking," appeared naked in public and exhibited "terrible outbursts of anger." Others were "violent in public" or "violent and destructive." A man, a 27-year-old clerk, got "into brawls after drinking omole."

This observation reflects a basic fact for these clients: their random aggression occurred while under the influence of omole or diamba. Frequently, the level of intoxication affected directly the nature and the intensity of the violence, with the excessively inebriated person causing more disturbance than the moderately drunk individual. In some instances, an etiology for chemical dependence was recorded: patients insisted that a difficult and stressful life event - perhaps the loss of a loved one, or failure at school, or a serious marital problem - was responsible for their violence and addiction.

The patterns of alcohol and drug abuse discerned in the inmates of Kissy hospital were confirmed in a study of drug problems in Sierra Leone, conducted in the mid-1980s. This analysis pointed to the predominance of young male offenders, noting that college and university students had become the largest group of drug users. Other elements in the population ranking high included motor vehicle drivers, farmers, and the unemployed. Marijuana was accessible and inexpensive, making it very popular.

Students assumed that smoking jamba facilitated their academic progress by increasing their intelligence and enhancing their skills for studying and taking examinations. In fact, cases were cited showing how marijuana abuse caused students to behave in bizarre ways, flirting with danger and death. While studying for a final exam, one student, for example, under the influence of marijuana felt that he could fly and jumped off the balcony of a dormitory. He escaped serious injury. Others, however, were not so fortunate. After a brief hospital stay, another student, a marijuana addict, died from internal bleeding, presumably the result of numerous falls occurring in states of delirium.

The report also observed that, along with marijuana, alcohol consumption had increased, particularly beer, palm wine, and omole. On the other hand, awareness of the dangers of datura stramonium or kube jarra had decreased its popularity. One incident dramatized its fatal hazards. Two students concocted a brew from kube jara, boiling its leaves and berry-like fruit. Within hours after drinking the substance, one student died, and the other student passed away a few days later, in Connaught Hospital. Still, the diminished appeal of datura stramonium remained incidental to the prevailing trend of increased abuse of drugs and alcohol by young men.

The report concluded that by the 1980s, chemical dependency, a dilemma emerging for twenty years, had become a serious public health problem in Sierra Leone.[2] This development formed part of a broader pattern occurring throughout sub-Saharan Africa in recent years. The findings of studies in Nigeria and Kenya, for example, echoed the results of investigations and reports on dependency in Sierra Leone, pointing to the relationships between drug use and other sociopathic behaviors. Drug dependency did not remain compartmentalized and segregated to the periphery of society; it fostered crime, family violence, and suicide, as well as social alienation and isolation.[3]

SCHIZOPHRENIA

In postcolonial Sierra Leone, the largest group of patients with a psychiatric designation suffered from schizophrenia. There were 265 cases - 182 males and 83 females - embracing several classifications. There were twenty paranoid type, eight catatonic, two schizo-affective, and one hebephrenic; other forms were labeled with general terms, namely, four acute schizophrenia, three chronic, one infantile, one incipient, three schizophrenic illness, and five schizoid personality. The rest of the group was diagnosed simply as being afflicted with schizophrenia.

Temne, Mende, and Krio formed the largest ethnic representations among the schizophrenics; some Limba and a few Sherbro, Foulah, and Kissi also were a part of the group. The majority of females were housewives and traders; the males were laborers, farmers, and prisoners, as well as seamen and teachers, and many were unemployed

The ages of the males and females ranged from 16 to 80, with the majority in their twenties and thirties. Most of the men were younger than the women. On the basis of this sample, schizophrenia in postcolonial Sierra Leone appears to have remained largely an affliction of young men in their twenties and middle-aged women above thirty.

One striking observation is the relatively rapid recovery, or general lack of chronicity, of many schizophrenic inmates. Over two-thirds of the group left the hospital within six months of admission; many returned to the community in less than three months. At the same time, a significant number of schizophrenics became long-term cases; over eighty remained in the asylum for a year or longer. A marked characteristics of these patients was repeated admissions. Many suffered relapses and were returned to the hospital on two or more occasions.

These general features of schizophrenics seem to be confirmed by studies of patients at mental hospitals throughout Africa. Reports across the continent reveal that schizophrenia was clearly the most common of all mental disorders.[4] And while some were crippled by it, many African schizophrenics achieved permanent recovery, a pattern evident also with other types of severe mental distress. Of course the availability of psychoactive medications by 1960 affected the manifestations of schizophrenic symptoms.

MANIC DEPRESSIVE PSYCHOSIS

Between 1960 and the 1980s, thirty-two patients, fifteen female and seventeen male, were designated as manic depressive cases. This group revealed demographic features generally similar to those of the schizophrenics. A major distinction, however, was that about the same number of women and men were afflicted with the disorder.

Of the manic depressives, those specifying an ethnic identity included nine Creole (Krio), two Sierra Leonean (Krio), one African (Krio), five Temne, two Mende, one Limba, one Yoruba, one Nigerian, and one Liberian. A few ages were recorded: the females averaged in their upper thirties, the males in their lower thirties.

Six of the women gave their occupations: there were two housewives, a clerk, and three traders. Eleven manic depressive men indicated their job identity: these included two traders, two clerks, a police officer, an army officer, a tailor, a civil servant, a laborer, a shoemaker, and a carpenter. The remaining fourteen persons were designated unemployed or without an occupation.

While the length of hospitalization of the manic depressives ranged from one day to ten years, only six inmates remained institutionalized for more than two years. Twelve persons were short-term cases and were released and sent home within six months or less. There were, however, eighteen patients with readmissions, notably five persons returning three times, two individuals having two relapses, and one patient suffering ten readmissions. A total of three patients died in the hospital. In general, this pattern follows the model of the schizophrenics: many patients returned to their communities, others had remissions, and a few became long-term hospital residents.

Most of these manic depressives displayed violent and belligerent behavior. One man was "dangerous to the entire community"; he "threatened lives" and was kept under police surveillance. A male Krio clerk terrorized children and attacked family members and neighbors. Another Sierra Leonean clerk was "always elated," and "dangerous with a knife"; he got "into fights after drinking omole." A woman, "emaciated and disorientated," attacked members of her household. And a Krio woman exhibited "difficult and violent" behavior at home; she drank and smoked excessively and wandered about the community "incurring fantastic expenses" by spending savings and trying to sell family property.

MANIA

Individuals designated as suffering from hypomania formed another group of severely distressed persons who engaged in threatening and disruptive behavior. In the postcolonial era, thirty patients, fourteen male and sixteen female, were identified with this disorder. In most instances, these hypomaniacs were out of control: a writing clerk destroyed furniture; a Mende man, during his "sudden outbursts of aggression," terrorized people; a Mende farmer went into government offices and caused disturbances; a female Susu trader ran after people with an axe; a seaman "became suddenly violent and aggressive and ran wild in the street threatening to harm others"; and another man "burned two houses."

Twelve of the hypomaniacs were Krio. Other ethnic groups represented included four Mende, one Temne, one Mandingo, one Sherbro, one Susu, one Limba, one Foulah, and one Hausa. Most of the women were traders or housewives; the occupational profile of the men embraced two farmers, a clerk, a cook, a motor driver, a seaman, a telephone operator, an apprentice druggist, and a stenographer. Nineteen of the cases were discharged within six months of admission; eleven remained in the hospital for a year or longer; there were eight inmates with one or more readmissions. These lengths of hospitalization conform to the general patterns of other types of severely disturbed inmates at Kissy and other African mental hospitals. Like the schizophrenics and the manic depressives, the majority of the hypomaniacs were released; some had relapses, and a few became chronic cases.

Among the Kissy clients in the independence period, there were still cases of mania, chronic mania, recurrent mania, recent mania, and acute mania. A Mende and a Nigerian, for example, were classified as mania cases. The Mende man, without friends or relatives, was characterized as "mentally deranged," a person who engaged in "nonsensical talk." He became a long-term hospital resident, remaining for over eight years. The Nigerian, a 40-year-old man who also made "irrelevant talk," had been in Sierra Leone for ten years. A single man without children, his house was destroyed by fire and his female companion left him, a disturbing event because he "spent lots of money" on her. After a week at Kissy, he was discharged, but he had two relapses, each of six weeks duration.

There were three chronic mania cases, one man and two women. The man was a married Krio cook from Bo who threatened and threw stones at people in the streets. His wife left him, and only one of his eight children survived. He held to a persistent delusion that he "killed a devil." After ten years of incarceration, he died in the Kissy hospital. The female chronic maniacs were both middle-aged Temne housewives who, after a brief stay in the mental institution, were sent to the King George VI Memorial Home. One woman died there; the other woman caused a "lot of trouble" and was shunted several times between the hospital and the home. A relative agreed to care for her.

The recurrent mania cases consisted of one woman and three men. The woman, a 29-year-old Krio housewife, had four readmissions. In each instance, after the "attack" subsided, she was discharged to the care of her husband. One of the males also experienced "recurrent attacks of uncontrollable behaviour." A stonemason for twenty-five years, the police arrested him on a charge of disorderly behavior. Released after a year and a half in the institution, he had a relapse and was readmitted for nine months.

In another case, that of a 42-year-old Krio schoolteacher, a divorce coupled with tense relations with professional colleagues contributed to the patient's disordered condition and return to the hospital. In the third male recurrent mania case, a troubled relationship led to violence and death. Claiming that his uncle "tormented him," the patient killed him, attempted suicide, and had several "attacks of violence." Sent to Kissy for observation, he absconded but was readmitted and eventually released to stand trial on a charge of murder.

Six recent mania cases, five men and one woman, were recorded. The woman was a 47-year-old Krio housewife who had a "history of mental disturbance." She stopped cars and displayed bizarre postures and grimaces. The four men were a Limba servant, a Mende store clerk, a Mende painter, and a Loko watchman. The servant was "excited and talkative," claiming that his father made him crazy. After two weeks in the hospital, he was discharged to the care of his father. The store clerk spent four years in the mental institution before he was released to his father. During his repeated mania attacks, he chased female staff members around the office. After a month's residence, the painter, a "restless, violent, and dirty" man, was sent home. He was readmitted for "disturbing the peace," and seven months later he absconded. The watchman, also a violent man, "threatened people" and started fights. Over a six-year period, he had eight readmissions to the asylum.

Seven men were labeled with acute mania. One patient, a Temne man who was called an exhibitionist, died within a year of institutionalization. A Limba farmer, designated a criminal lunatic, became a good worker in the hospital and remained for over nine years. Two other men were long-term inmates: a Temne farmer, a single man with a history of domestic violence, was maintained for three years; and a Foulah trader, who enjoyed staying in the hospital, was kept for three years.

Three acute maniacs were short-term cases: a Loko trader stayed for a month; although "wild on admission," he may simply have drunk too much palm wine. The second person was a Mende watchmaker who "rushed about in the nude;" after spending a week at Kissy, his friends promised to care for him. And a student at Njala University, subject to bouts of insomnia, ran around singing and shouting and stayed at Kissy for a month.

MISCELLANEOUS CASES

Nine patients formed a mélange of psychiatric cases. Acute psychosis was ascribed to a Limba carpenter who ran around naked. He was discharged and readmitted, returning to the hospital with his pockets full of stones. Two years later he was released on trial to the care of his brother. A middle-aged, married Krio prison worker was designated an acute paranoid delusionary. One night he plunged into a stream, poured a bucket of water over his head, and asked his wife to shave him, asserting that "a Muslim ceremony" would "be performed on him." The next day he ran out into the street, shouting and tearing his clothes, claiming that all his possessions belonged to others. After seven days at Kissy, he was discharged to the outpatient clinic, and, was later readmitted to the asylum for two weeks.

Compulsive obsessional was the psychiatric term given to a 44-year-old Krio civil servant. Hospitalized for thirty days, he too, on occasion, ran naked in the streets. More often, he sulked and remained frustrated over his inability to stop drinking and taking drugs. Another 44-year-old Krio, a married freight clerk suffering from chronic melancholia, lived "in a world of his own," refusing to communicate or answer questions. Eighteen months of hospitalization did not cure him; his condition deteriorated, and he died in the facility.

Delusional insanity was applied to a 34-year-old Krio evangelist with three admissions to the hospital. Immature personality was attributed to a 21-year-old Yoruba woman. While she received numerous weekend furloughs, she remained a patient for over five years. A Krio cook, a woman identified with anxiety neurosis, was obsessed with drinking water. After spending sixty days at Kissy, she was sent home to the care of her daughters. Hypertension was applied to a woman suffering from devastating life events - the deaths of her husband and nine of her ten children. Discharged after seven days, she could not care for herself and was readmitted for six weeks. And a 19-year-old Krio police officer was observed for twenty-four hours and discharged; he had a hysterical reaction to attacks of dizziness.

GPI AND SENILITY

Another group of nine patients, two women and seven men, consisted of middle-aged and elderly GPI cases. As in the earlier period, these were instances of neurosyphilis. One of the women, a 58-year-old Mende trader who experienced rapid mood changes, died three months after admission. The other woman was a Krio without relatives or friends. One male Temne trader who talked "nonsense for a year" was also a long-term resident. Two of the male GPI patients died in the hospital: a Temne farmer with elephantiasis of the scrotum, and a man who constantly laughed and rolled on the ground. The remaining three males were sent to the memorial home: a Krio who believed that cannibals were chasing him, a "moody" man from the French Cameroons, and a "confused and deluded" Temne charged with unlawful assault.

Six patients, two men and four women, received psychiatric designations related to advanced age. A 60-year-old single, unemployed man, "a destructive and abusive" person, was a dementia case. He spent four years in the hospital and was discharged to the care of his nephew. A Temne farmer, suffering from senile psychosis, held bewildering delusions of grandeur. Lacking initiative, he could not care for himself and became a permanent hospital resident. A Temne woman, a case of senile confusion, assumed that the mental hospital was a mosque. She remained cheerful and foolish and was taken to the memorial home. The label of senile dementia was assigned to three women. A disoriented Temne woman, a beggar deserted by her husband

and son, was maintained in the hospital for two years and died. Another woman without family support - an impoverished son could not look after her - was kept at the memorial home. And an 84-year-old housewife, who, many years earlier had disturbed the peace and beaten up little children, died after a long residence in the asylum.

PUERPERAL PSYCHOSIS

In the colonial era, only one patient, a 34-year-old Limba woman, suffered from peurperal insanity. At Connaught Hospital in Freetown, she shouted and made noises without cause and tried to jump out of a window. After three days at Kissy, she became quiet, wanted to see her baby, and was discharged to the care of her husband.[5] After 1960, puerperal psychosis affected twenty women admitted to Kissy hospital: there were eleven housewives and a nurse, along with eight women listed without an occupation. Only seven gave an ethnic identity: three Krio, two Temne, one Limba, and one Nigerian.

In some traditional African societies, a psychiatric illness during the puerperium might indicate infidelity of the mother during pregnancy. Or, more often, it was blamed on sorcery, and therefore a traditional healer accepted the responsibility to neutralize and remove any threat to the sick person. At Kissy hospital, and other African mental institutions, women with postpartum psychoses were treated with drugs and, until the end of the 1970s, ECT - electroconvulsive therapy. When a patient showed no improvement, ECT was discontinued.

The length of hospitalization for the twenty patients ranged from two days to eight months; fourteen inmates were sent home within three months. Such a favorable prognosis for the group was dampened by the six clients who had one or more readmissions.

In most instances, symptoms appeared within two weeks following delivery. One woman, a week after the birth of her child, became dumb and refused to eat. Many of these women displayed apathy, insomnia, and withdrawal, coupled with occasional "outbursts of restlessness" or destructive and disorderly activity. Some patients appeared mentally defective. Paranoid delusions and hallucinations were common.

One mother rejected the infant and had to be restrained by family members. In this situation, ECT "very much improved" her condition, and she returned home. In another case, the mother killed the child. She threw the baby in a toilet; after three weeks at Kissy, she was discharged to the care of the police. An experience of unusual social and psychological stress precipitated one mother's disturbed conduct: while she felt sad over the death of her baby, a violent quarrel with her husband, during which he burned her clothes, led her to run naked in the street. She spent two days in the hospital and absconded.

EPILEPSY AND MENTAL RETARDATION

During the postcolonial era, five epileptics - two women and three men - and sixteen mentally retarded persons - four women and twelve men - were sent to Kissy hospital. The epileptics were a young group: the females were 14 to 20; two men were 16 and 17, and the third male was described as "a well-nourished young man." One of the males remained institutionalized for four years. After a brief stay in the hospital, the other epileptics were sent back to relatives or local communities. Two of the males exhibited violent and self-destructive conduct.

In the mentally retarded group, two clients, a 26-year-old woman and a 16-year-old Kissy village boy, were also designated as epileptics. The woman had several readmissions to the hospital. According to the case report, she was "always a problem child." She left school and could not master dressmaking or typing skills. At home, her mother could not cope with her destructive behavior. A cycle of hope and despair ensued: after a stay in the hospital, the daughter returned home, but soon she became unruly and was sent back to the institution. A few weeks later, the same pattern of events resumed.

The Kissy boy, specified mentally deficient, was an equally difficult patient, but in a different way. Physically handicapped, he was unable to care for himself. He had daily fits and could not talk. Relatives, however, agreed to look after him.

Six of the mentally retarded inmates also received psychiatric labels: there were three schizophrenics, a manic depressive, a depressive and a GPI. The schizophrenics were long-term residents: a Sierra Leonean farmer, a hoarder of rubbish, laughed giggled, and smiled "for no apparent reason." He received twelve electroconvulsive treatments without "the slightest change" and remained in the hospital for over eight years. A 28-year-old Temne steward, tagged feeble-minded, talked nonsense and became aggressive when thwarted by any event. He was maintained for over five years.

A 24-year-old single mentally deficient woman was called "an old case of schizophrenia." Her record states that she "roams the streets of Freetown at some ungodly hours of the night in a very wretched and uncared for and unsightly manner." The one manic depressive patient was discharged, against medical advice, to his relatives within a week of admission. After three years at Kissy, the depressive, a Temne tailor with a history of violence, was removed to his sister's home.

The GPI case, a Mende man, spent eight months in the institution and returned, on trial, to his home in the provinces, where a daughter reluctantly accepted responsibility for him. Another dual designation, "mentally deficient and deranged," was assigned to a 47-year-old Krio stonemason, a violent man who attacked family members. After a year and four months, he died in the hospital. A Kuranko man, a hospital resident of nearly two years who resented discipline and hoarded rubbish, also died in the facility. The youngest case of retardation, a 12-year-old girl, was returned to her mother after four months. A case of murder and suicide, a Mende man, was kept in the hospital for an unspecified length of time. Two other men also became institutionalized: a 25-year-old African for six years, and a 23-year-old house servant for twenty-three years.

The remaining patients in this group, a 25-year-old Krio woman and a Mende carpenter, both received electroconvulsive treatment, but "without noticeable benefit." Although the woman was described as "completely disoriented," "immature," and "underdeveloped," she was allowed, on occasion, weekend furloughs. And the carpenter, after five weeks, was moved to the memorial home.

A demographic survey of the retarded group reveals that no occupations were assigned to the women, while the men included a carpenter, a tailor, a farmer, a house servant, a steward, and a stonemason. The ethnic composition included five Krio, three Mende, two Temne, and one Kuranko.

Like the epileptics, this was a relatively young group: the oldest person was 47, the youngest 12, with the average age around 25. The length of hospitalization varied from one week to twenty-three years, and most of the inmates became long-term residents. Still, the administration made efforts to arrange for home care.

SUICIDE

Throughout the 1980s, suicide remained a minor psychiatric problem. Its relatively low incidence may be attributed to the continuing lack of a sense of personal guilt among the populace, traditional taboos against it, and the fact that it is illegal. Between 1960 and the 1980s, sixty-two patients at Kissy hospital, seventeen females and forty-five males, were associated with suicide. From this group, those women indicating an occupation included eight housewives, a student, and an assistant bookbinder. Among the men, there were four farmers, three traders, two schoolteachers, a laborer, a mechanic, a freight clerk, a tailor, a fisherman, a seaman, a student, a policeman, a prisoner, a government printer, a driver, a businessman, and two unemployed.

The ethnic groups specified were two foreigners, a Nigerian and a Ghanaian, three African (Krio), one Sierra Leonean (Krio), five Creole (Krio), eight Mende, five Temne, one Limba, one Syrian, and one Sherbro. On the basis of those who gave a birthdate, the age pattern for the parasuicides followed the model for most types of mental illness in Sierra Leone: the men were younger than the women; they averaged in their twenties, the women in their thirties. The spread of ages ranged from 16 to 50 for males and 22 to 50 for females.

The methods of attempted suicide did not vary significantly between the sexes. In thirty-two cases, the specifics of self-destruction were noted: the most frequent method was cutting one's throat - the way chosen by nine males and five females. A man and a woman jumped from a building; hanging was attempted by a man and a woman; two men and a woman took an overdose of sleeping tablets; a woman asked God to kill her; three men tried drowning; varied self-inflicted wounds were made by a woman and two men; a 16-year-old boy chewed razor blades; a man set fire to a mattress and blocked all ventilation into the room; a woman threw herself in front of a moving vehicle; and a man drank carbolic acid and kerosene. The records of the thirty other parasuicides noted only that the client "tried to commit suicide," had "attempted suicide," or was "suicidal."

Numerous reasons were given for attempted self-murder. Supernatural intervention impelled six people to consider suicide. Three men and a woman indicated that "a devil" or "the devils" told them to self-destruct; two women were convinced that juju, or witchcraft, contributed to their parasuicide. In other cases, difficult and emotionally painful relationships constituted a precipitating factor: to escape from a nagging wife, a husband tried to end his life; one man's girlfriend was "planning to desert him"; a wife felt depressed over her husband's lack of interest in her; a young man became distraught over his mother's hostility toward his girlfriend; a bitter quarrel with his mother led a son to attempt to drown himself. A series of devastating events, namely, the deaths of her father, husband, and child, contributed to one woman's effort to kill herself. Alcoholism was associated with one female and three male parasuicides. Social and emotional isolation played a major role in the attempted suicide of two men: a lonely Nigerian traveling businessman who was mistaken for a thief and beaten up and abandoned, and a homeless, insecure man who slept on church steps.

With other persons, parasuicide may have been a manifestation of the individual's general psychosis. Twenty-five patients from this group had psychiatric designations as follows: five schizophrenia, four male and one female; one male schizophrenia paranoid type; one male hypomania; one male recent mania; one male recurrent mania; one male infantile psychopathic; one male mentally retarded; one male manic depressive; one male chronic melancholia; one female recent depression; one male acute depression; and ten depressive illness, eight male and two female.

This characterization of a group of parasuicides in Sierra Leone conforms largely to studies of suicide and parasuicide in other parts of Africa. Reports from Kenya, Ethiopia, and Nigeria reveal the most obvious similarity: like in Sierra Leone, these countries have a low incidence of self-destruction. Very few elderly persons are involved; the rate is highest in the age group 19 to 30 years. In Nigeria, like Sierra Leone, many more men than women attempt suicide. On the other hand, the studies of Ethiopian and Kenyan patients show no significant sex difference. In contrast to Sierra Leone, poisoning is the preferred method in Kenya, and hanging the most frequent mode in Ethiopia and Nigeria. Factors precipitating parasuicide show similarity across these countries, yet vary from region to region.

In the Nairobi, Kenya study, most of the attempted suicides constituted a reaction to a stressful situation, notably the breakup of a romantic affair, domestic quarrels, marital disharmony, and fear of having a fatal disease. The motives for suicide revealed in the Ethiopian and Nigerian studies had a somatic or medical nature as well as some social factor, and related more closely to those of the Sierra Leone group. There was psychosis or evidence of serious mental illness in numerous instances, and in other cases, there were indications of such social and psychological problems as alcohol abuse, personal estrangement, marriage conflict, witchcraft, and bereavement.[6]

DEPRESSION

In Sierra Leone between 1960 and the 1980s, sixty-nine patients entered Kissy hospital - twenty-seven male and forty-two female - suffering from depression. The psychiatric breakdown included thirty-one depressive illness, twenty-three depression, two acute depression, three agitated depression, one retarded depression, two recent depression, one recurrent depression, one endogenuous depression, one reactive depression, one depressive psychopath, one depressive features, and one depressive state.

Forty-three persons from this group designated occupations. Among the women, there were nineteen housewives, a farmer, a nurse, a trader, a typist, a student, and a cook; among the men, there were three farmers, a police corporal, a veterinarian assistant, a mason, a laborer, three traders, a fisherman, a part-time artist, a watchmaker, a carpenter, a post-office accountant, and three unemployed.

The ethnic makeup of thirty-five members of the group of depressive cases embraced nine Temne, two Mende, two Loko, one Kissi, one Kroo, one Foulah, two Yoruba, nine African (Krio), two Sierra Leonean (Krio), and six Creole (Krio). Ages averaged in the late twenties for men and the late thirties for the women.

The length of hospitalization of most depressives was under six months; eight patients remained for more than a year, with the longest staying five years and two months. There were twenty-one readmissions, including eight multiple readmissions. Two inmates were sent to the King George VI Memorial Home; and three died in the hospital.

The case records are replete with statements depicting the mood and physical appearance of these inmates. In most instances, the traditional and popular characterization of the depressive was used. The patients was described as "severely depressed," or "agitated and depressed," or "withdrawn and depressed, or it was said that the inmate "looks and feels depressed." A suicidal tendency was apparent in twelve cases, nine males and three females.

Domestic or marital trouble was, according to the hospital records, the cause of several depressions. A housewife, for example, was disturbed that her frequent quarrels with her husband had become a topic of neighborhood gossip. Another woman was distraught over her husband's infidelity. A 35-year-old single African woman was depressed over the retraction of a marriage proposal. A withdrawn and sad appearance enveloped a woman abandoned by her husband, as well as a wife who felt threatened by her husband's new, young wife.

Grief over the death of a family member, notably a wife or a husband, contributed to the depression of other inmates. An accident emotionally jarred a Kroo housewife: a hot lamp fell on her child's stomach; she assumed responsibility for the incident and became depressed when the infant's abdomen did not quickly heal.

With some patients there were frequent somatic complaints: a Temne man talked about "things crawling" on his skin, and an African housewife claimed that a "sickness wandered all over her body." Another woman said that "something in her chest goes up her throat and then back to the abdomen"; it bit the back of her throat, she asserted, and returned to her heart. Such remarks were accompanied by hypochondriacal symptoms, as well as paranoid delusions or auditory hallucinations. And a few cases of depression stemmed from drug and alcohol abuse.

The pattern of depressive illness in Sierra Leone followed largely the trend of this disorder in other parts of Africa. While cases of melancholia were evident, the diagnosis of depression in Africans, until the 1950s, was nonexistent or very rare. Accounts of medical practitioners, based on mental hospital or general hospital clients in South Africa, Kenya, and the Gold Coast, were in general agreement: depression was rare among Africans; when occurring, it was mild and short-lived; and suicide and self-denigration, elements in the depressions of European psychotics, were unusual.[7] In 1936, H. L. Gordon, reporting on admissions to Mathare Hospital in Kenya, observed that an exp'anation for the paucity of African depressives was not possible ⌐ecause "we are too ignorant of the normal native mind."[8]

About twenty years later, the pattern changed. During the African independence era, beginning in 1957 with the emergence of Ghana, clinicians found higher rates of depression. This finding may be attributed to such factors as a greater sensitivity to the condition, an increased incidence of depression, and larger numbers of indigenous personnel capable of detecting the disorder.

A common theme emerged from the reports: while the rates of depression in Africa were now assumed to be as high as those of other cultures, the form and content of African depression differed significantly from the European model. Physicians held that somatic rather than psychological symptoms masked depression in African patients. These indications might include appetite disturbances, sleep disorders, or bodily complaints such as weakness, fatigue, headaches, and sensations of burning in the head or other parts of the body. Along with somaticism and hypochondriasis, other types of symptoms peculiar to African depression might include paranoid delusions, auditory hallucinations, and sexual impotence.

Recent studies indicate that somatic symptoms have been complemented with expressions of sadness and self-depreciation, particularly among women who feel useless or helpless and assume that they no longer have a meaningful role. Such feelings were present among the housewives from the group of Sierra Leone depressives. The findings also suggest that the more educated, individualistic, and Westernized patients show the common or classical indications of depression, succumbing to the types found in Europe and North America.[9] Cultural differences, however, do prevail. A comparison of the characteristics of depressives in the United Kingdom and in Nigeria revealed that certain behavior patterns were culturally determined. While a mood of dejection was evident in both samples, there were distinctions: the prevalence of somatic symptoms ranked low in the London group, while among Benin patients, guilt and suicidal ideas remained uncommon.[10]

An additional factor complicating the analysis of depression in Africa is the culture's prevailing view of illness and disease, which attributes sickness to forces outside of the individual - that is, to the contrivance of witches, malevolent forces, or jealous associates. A study of a group of West African depressives demonstrated that 20 percent of the sample had delusions and hallucinations related to witchcraft.[11] The wide acceptance of sorcery has undercut and depreciated the value of a physician or psychiatrist, frustrating efforts at detecting and monitoring depressive illness. A person distressed and overwrought by the apparent machinations of a wizard would not consult a psychiatrist for help or solace. The sick individual would look for advice and direction from a traditional healer, someone sensitive to popular beliefs about the nature of madness and disease. This type of mental health care has remained most apparent in rural areas, where depressives attend religious healing ceremonies and are treated at native shrines.[12]

WITCHCRAFT

Between 1960 and the 1980s, witchcraft illusions were the primary affections of eighty-eight patients - forty women and forty-eight men - at Kissy hospital. This was a group largely of chronic and severe cases of mental disorder; many were readmissions. Over 65 percent were long-term cases, hospitalized for over six months. Of this number, over 50 percent were institutionalized for one year or longer.

Forty-five persons received no psychiatric designation; twenty-two were labeled with schizophrenia. Other diagnoses included four mania, five depressive illness, five alcoholic psychosis, one GPI, one mental retardation, two psychopath, one senile dementia, one suicidal, and one immature personality.

The group had a diverse makeup consisting of eleven African (Krio), one Creole (Krio), eight Mende, eight Temne, three Susu, two Yalunka, one Joloff, one Loko, one Sherbro, one Mandingo, one Yoruba, and one Nigerian.

The ages ranged from 16 to 58, with the majority of the men averaging in their late twenties, and the women in their mid- and late thirties. Occupationally, the group consisted largely of housewives, traders, and farmers, along with some unemployed, a few prisoners, and students, and people holding service-related jobs.

A few people from this group believed themselves devils or witches. A farmer, for example, claimed that he was "a devil with magical power" who could do anything in the world. A woman confessed: "I am a witch." This condition gave her no advantage since, she observed, her husband had transformed her previously "into an animal." Some patients, seeking protection from a devil or a witch, took varied security measures: one man wore a cord around his neck, a 31-year-old Temne man sacrificed a sheep to protect him from "a devil in the family."

The most striking kinds of illusions from this group relate to visual perceptions of devils and machinations of evil spirits controlling humans. Many of the patients admitted seeing a devil. It might take the form of "a female devil with her head cut off," a "white devil woman," a "black devil," or a "tall devil." Frequently, there were several demons: when alone, for example, a woman "saw devils," a man envisioned "devils and baboons were chasing him," and one inmate saw "devils at night" and assumed that all the patients in the hospital were evil-doers.

On occasion, some clients asserted that devils spoke to them. Also, many members of this group felt manipulated by witches or devils. There were general complaints: the devil or devils "influenced" or "disturbed" or "harassed" a patient.

More often, the delusion caused a specific and frightening event, accompanied by a feeling of terror. Two young women, for example, were convinced that a devil had raped them. Others insisted that devils had instructed them to kill themselves. A Temne housewife said that devils told her "to kill and wash herself in the victim's blood." A particularly gruesome case involved a young man who claimed that a devil told him to self-destruct by chewing and swallowing razor blades. Another man assumed that his 1-year-old son had been transformed into a devil; to stop the evil one, he picked up a machete and split the child's head. Two young men believed that their girlfriends had been changed into witches, and now were tormenting their former lovers.

The machinations of a devil or a witch were often used to explain poor health, an unfortunate happening, or sexual troubles. A devil was held responsible, for example, for a person's insanity, or a devil's doings were felt to have led to the incarceration of a patient in the mental hospital. To a Krio housemaid, an evil spirit had "put something in her head," making her mentally ill. While washing clothes, a woman accidently dropped her baby; she attributed the child's fall and subsequent crying to the work of a devil. A few young women complained that a witch had made them barren, incapable of having a child. And "powerful devils" visited an inmate at night, informing him that a witch had destroyed his genitals and was "eating the inside of his mouth."

DELUSIONS

Along with witchcraft preoccupations, other types of delusions were evident among Kissy patients. Visions of grandeur, secular and religious, figured prominently in the mental makeup of sixty-three hospital inmates - 50 men and 13 women. Some of the recorded assertions of these patients were quite general: a person was "wealthy," had "money," or "plenty of money." In other cases, more specific claims were made: a 46-year-old Susu trader insisted that he owned "4,000 cars and lorries and tons of money"; a Temne farmer, suffering from senile psychosis, had "90 bags of silver coins and 20 bags of paperback notes"; a Temne woman believed that she owned the entire country.

In addition to delusions of property and money, some inmates saw themselves elevated to positions of power and high responsibility. Several believed that they were paramount chiefs. A laborer said that he was "a mighty power with an all seeing eye." There were two kings of England, a king and owner of Freetown, a queen of England, two queens, a queen of queens, a president of Ghana, a president of Liberia, three presidents of Sierra Leone, the wife of the president of Sierra Leone, and assorted government officials and relatives of important persons in Sierra Leone and the United Kingdom.

Many of the delusions from this group were religious. An unemployed man said that he was "a messenger of God." Another man claimed: "I am in contact with God. He sends me messages." Quite often, patients felt that a special spiritual mission had been assigned to them. A Mandingo laborer heard the voice of God, "telling him to do good and tell the truth." A 34-year-old Krio man believed that God had selected him "to cure the ways of Man." A Temne farmer, a schizophrenic, viewed himself as "the last prophet sent by God to preach his Gospel." Several patients assumed an even more exalted position: the identity of Jesus Christ was taken by four inmates, and two others said that they were God. A Temne farmer announced: "I am Mohammed." A Temne woman proclaimed that "the prophet Mohammed" had "put her in charge of the world."

In a few instances, a religious delusion justified a dastardly act or thought. A 42-year-old farmer said that God told him to attack and rape women. A housewife, subject to spells of weeping, confessed that "God advised her to kill a relative."

There were some unique cases of delusion. One man, for example, a paranoid schizophrenic, who spent a year in the hospital, claimed that "space magicians" controlled his behavior, notably by forcing his participation in an attempted coup in Guinea. The United Nations, he said, was investigating the matter. He believed further that all his thoughts were the ideas of others imposed on him and that "magical mirrors" were being utilized to watch him.

In another case, a young man subject to a fixed delusion carried a letter alerting people to his special condition. The letter was addressed "To the World at Large" and noted that this person was "unfortunately unbalanced in mind," the result of losing all his money. He aspired "to become the next Prime Minister, without a general election." And the letter ended with the observation that he was "harmless but he should be treated with caution and sympathy."

The occupations of this group of delusionaries included mostly traders and housewives among the women, and farmers, laborers, traders, prisoners, and the unemployed among the men. This was an older cluster of inmates, with the men averaging in their mid-thirties. Only four women specified ages; these were 18, 25, 37, and 41. Hospitalization was of relatively long duration, with the majority classified as long-term patients, residing in the hospital for over nine months. Twenty-five persons remained longer than one year.

Thirty-two patients received no psychiatric designation; the diagnoses for the others included eighteen schizophrenia, eight hypomania, three manic depressive, one senile psychosis, one delusional insanity, three alcoholic psychosis, and two compulsive obsessional (drug addiction). No GPI patients were in this group, a pertinent fact considering that grandiose delusions represent an outstanding symptom of GPI.

Individuals with a recorded ethnic identity included nine Temne, three Mende, four Creole (Krio), two Sierra Leonean (Krio), one Liberated African (Krio), six African (Krio), one Mandingo, one Sherbro, one Yoruba, one Liberian, and one Indian.

CONFUSIONAL STATES

The psychiatric designation confusional state was assigned to seven patients, five men and two women. One of the women, for example, had fallen down, suffering a cut lip and head injury. Initially, she was confused and aggressive. After two days at Kissy, she became quiet and orderly, "fully accessible," and was discharged. A Temne farmer, a nudist, complained about dizziness and a swollen foot. Within a week, he was released to the care of his wife. A Kroo man, inaccessible and violent on admission, and in poor health, became physically weak and wasted and died within five months, of bilateral pneumonia. In another fatality, an African blacksmith, troublesome and disoriented, suffering from hypertension and abdominal pain, died in three weeks, the apparent victim of a vascular accident. Another confusional state patient was a Nigerian trader who became a public nuisance: he jumped into a car and refused to leave, he picked quarrels for no apparent reason, and he fought with a man. After two months at Kissy, he was repatriated to Nigeria.

Two other cases included an emotionally unstable Foulah tailor who alternately laughed and cried and displayed "extremely foolish," "rambling" behavior. After six weeks he was discharged to the care of his relatives. And an elderly Limba woman, "a harmless destitute," was sent to the memorial home. Although she occasionally complained about being "sick all over her body," she remained largely inaccessible and spoke nonsense. Three years after admission, she died at Connaught Hospital.

NONDESIGNATED CASES

Out of the postcolonial pool of patients, 1,083 persons - 738 men and 345 women - received no psychiatric designation. The largest percentage of males was under the age of 30; the highest percentage of women was over 30. The ages and marital status of the group support epidemiological data from colonial Sierra Leone, as well as from other societies, notably in Europe and North America. As in the preindependence period, single young men and middle-aged married women formed a large portion of Kissy hospital clientele, a characteristic also disclosed in studies of mental patients in other parts of the world.

Patients specifying an ethnic identity included the following: seventy-six Mende, fifty-six Temne, thirty-one Creole (Krio), eleven African (Krio), eight Sierra Leonean (Krio), four Foulah, twenty-two Susu, nineteen Limba, six Sherbro, two Kroo, six Loko, one Kuranko, one Yalunka, five Mandingo, one Fanti, one Yoruba, seven Nigerian, two Gambian, three Liberian, five Guinean, two Ghanaian, three Lebanese, one Syrian, and two Indian.

A changing religious pattern was a new demographic feature of the nondesignates. In the colonial era, Christianity was the most common religious affiliation of Kissy patients. Beginning in the 1960s, while Christianity remained the choice of many clients, increasingly it was supplanted by Islam. Two hundred and sixteen of the nondesignates indicated a religious preference: 137 chose the Muslim faith, 66 Christianity, 7 Roman Catholic, 1 Methodist, and 5 were labeled pagans.

The occupational status of the nonspecified cases was equally significant. Among males and females, a wide assortment of vocations were represented. For the men, these included blacksmith, tinsmith, butcher, baker, watch repairer, shoemaker, messenger, time keeper, artisan, boatman, barber, mattress mover, watchman, wireman, fitter, prison warder, as well as such professional positions as nurse, social worker, surveyor, sales manager, technician, and barrister. Occupations with more than one representative from this group included teacher, mason, soldier, cook, fisherman, farmer, student, clerk, seaman, police constable, driver, laborer, security guard, steward, porter, motor mechanic, palm-wine tapper, carpenter, and civil servant. The largest number of men, however, was outside the occupational system: prisoners and the unemployed constituted a major part of the nondesignated male inmates.

For the women, the jobs embraced fishmonger, dressmaker, seamstress, trader, cook, housenurse, midwife, housemaid, cleaner, hospital worker, ward attendant, student, clerk, secretary, social worker, nurse, librarian, and typist. While some prisoners and the unemployed were female, a large segment of women identified themselves as housewives.

Most of the nonspecified clients were short-term patients, residing in the hospital for less than ninety days. A significant number absconded, especially during the first week of institutionalization. For instance, out of a sample of eighty-two inmates who left the hospital within seven days, twenty-eight had escaped. Some patients were returned to prison or sent to the memorial home.

Only a few inmates from the entire group of nondesignates died in the hospital. The health of the person, more than any other variable, determined the timing of an individual's death. Two patients, for example, in poor condition, died shortly after entering the hospital; other inmates, in good physical shape, remained for decades, passing away thirty years later. In some cases, gender determined the length of stay, with many males discharged within sixty days of admission, and females maintained for ninety days or longer.

While Freetown and its environs remained the major source of these unclassified patients, clients did come, often with a police escort, from the smaller urban areas in other parts of the country, notably from Bo, Kambia, Kenema, Kailahun, Makeni, Moyamba, and Sefadu. As earlier, under the certificate of emergency system, an individual could be sent to Kissy Mental Hospital for an observation period ranging from a few days to a few weeks. The document specified the reasons for temporary incarceration.

A large number of the nondesignated patients were hospitalized for committing some public disturbance or violent act. For example, a soldier from the military barracks was "violent whilst on duty." A man from Moyamba was "violent and a nuisance." A Mende woman was described as "a menace to the town"; another woman was "uncontrollable at home," she "accosts people and stones houses." A man in Freetown, with a "history of violence," was "violent and aggressive towards people in the streets." A man sent from Makeni Hospital claimed that "his head turns"; the medical officer observed that he "gets wild and goes into the bush and threatens people with a machete." A teacher, under the influence of "excessive drinking," exhibited "terrible outbursts of anger"; he "appeared naked in public, shouting and throwing stones at the school compound."

This was not an isolated case. There were numerous instances of alcohol and drug abuse among the unclassified cases and most of these patients displayed some form of aggressive behavior. A chronic alcoholic, admitted and discharged several times, destroyed property and attacked his wife and children, as well as people in the streets. In an intoxicated state, a young man from Makeni roamed the streets, threatening people with a knife. Several patients were referred to as "a problem drinker," or "a drug addict." Invariably, they were described as being "antagonistic," or "negativistic," or "violent and aggressive" at home or in public. Such conduct often demanded police intervention.

A very large percentage of the unclassified patients were criminal offenders. While the most frequent charges were disorderly behavior, threatening remarks, and malicious damage, some patients were guilty of assault, indecent exposure, housebreaking, burglary, larceny, unlawful possession of an offensive weapon, attempted suicide, and, in a few cases, arson and murder. In these matters, the medical or police officer specified the need for a period of observation at Kissy in order to determine the sanity of the offending person.

Along with their criminal actions, such individuals did exhibit varied indications of mental distress, either during or after apprehension by the authorities. A woman from Waterloo, charged with disorderly behavior, was "incoherent and had no insight"; a housewife guilty of larceny engaged in "senseless conversation."

One person "seems to be insane"; others were tagged "inaccessible," or "impossible to interview," "restless and confused," or "abusive and uncooperative." Some patients complained of delusions and visual hallucinations.

While a few of these individuals absconded, most recovered and were released to the police. A curt notation was placed on the case record: "Fit to stand trial." On occasion, a person committing a sensational crime went to the mental hospital. A man who hacked a woman with a machete confessed to the act and turned himself over to the police. After spending two months at Kissy, he was transferred to the prison. The medical officer commented: "Absolutely no evidence whatsoever of any psychiatric impairment or mental illness."

In addition to recent offenders, long-term prisoners constituted another segment of the unclassified. Here, the abnormal behavior of the convict led to his transfer to Kissy. There were several instances of persons singing and shouting in their cells, seemingly oblivious to their surroundings. Numerous cases involved prisoners who refused to wear clothes. A woman, sentenced for disorderly behavior, repeatedly tore off her clothes, insisting that she remain nude. Some convicts were not violent. A man was shunted between prison and asylum several times because of his withdrawn and severely depressed conduct. A more typical case dealt with a 25-year-old single man, incarcerated for larceny. He wrote on walls, engaged in filthy practices, fought with others, and generally was "boisterous and violent." Another larceny case was a 43-year-old single man who was maintained for thirty-six years in the mental hospital. He died in the memorial home. This was a rare case. Most long-term convicts were short-term mental patients; they recovered and went back to prison, staying only a few days or weeks at Kissy.

TRANSIENT PSYCHOSIS

While the unclassified patients from 1960 through the 1980s represented a diverse body of people, the majority were poor, young, single males. Some were habituated to omole and diamba; many were unemployed. Many were found guilty of committing a violent act, and were sent to prison or the mental hospital for a few weeks or months. This type of patient, with or without chemical dependence, was also prevalent in colonial Sierra Leone and equally evident in other African countries.

Various medical authorities have focused attention on the behavior patterns as well as the large numbers of unclassified inmates in African mental hospitals. In 1956, for example, over a six-month period, 304 patients were admitted to Mulago Mental Hospital in Kampala, Uganda; 57 persons received a diagnosis, 247 remained unclassified. These inmates exhibited symptoms and behavior that were difficult to diagnose, a situation apparent in other areas of East Africa, notably Kenya, along with places in West Africa, including Nigeria, Ghana, and Guinea.[13]

This condition received numerous labels: transient psychosis remained the most generally accepted term. Other designations included psychosis-like state, periodic psychosis, fear psychosis, atypical psychosis, atypical paranoid psychosis, and frenzied anxiety. Occasionally, a nineteenth century term, hysterical psychosis, appeared in the literature. In Francophone Africa, the designation bouffées delirantes was applied widely; here medical observers maintained that the condition could be applied to over 30 percent of African psychoses.

The reports from these various authorities outlined several fluctuating syndromes, the most common involving delusions and hallucinations, as well as episodes of excitement and confusion that frequently led to violence. A good prognosis followed: this was a short-term disorder. The psychotic confusional state passed, and the condition cleared up completely after a few weeks or months.

The etiology of the malady has aroused much concern and speculation. Medical authorities have pointed to varied organic factors that could adversely affect the central nervous system, notably syphilis, malaria, and meningo-encephalitis, as well as parasitic infestations and pulmonary infections. General malnutrition combined with minor illness might produce psychotic symptoms. The same behavior could be produced by climate-related vicissitudes such as heat stroke and rapid dehydration. Drug addiction, the inadvertent poisoning and administration of traditional medicines or pharmaceuticals, and some witchcraft practices can induce acute psychotic states. Psychiatrists and anthropologists have made extensive commentaries on the intense anxiety states caused by the fear of bewitchment. Others point to the stresses created by rapid social changes, notably urbanization, the shift from communalism to individualism, and the identity crisis of the person caught between traditional African culture and the ways of the West. Indeed, transient psychoses seem most prevalent in Third World cultures undergoing rapid alternation.[14]

This cultural conflict and stress was exacerbated further by the economic downturn occurring across Africa, and in Sierra Leone, during the 1970s and 1980s. The majority of patients at Kissy Mental Hospital, both unclassified and in all categories of illness, came from the bottom rungs of society, a pattern also evident in mental institutions in the developed world. Toward the end of the twentieth century, however, in the sub-Saharan region, the economically troubled times expanded the numbers of identifiably poor people, bringing new inmates into the hospital and undercutting its effectiveness. Significantly, a growing hostility toward the mad poor became apparent; the insane poor became undesirables. Like beggars, they were seen as parasites and nuisances to be shunted away from the wider community and incarcerated.

NOTES

1. This chapter rests on an examination of the case records of patients admitted to Kissy Mental Hospital between 1960 and the 1980s. The exact cut-off point varied with the individual; some cases extended into the 1980s, some did not. In the interests of protecting the rights and preserving the anonymity of clients, it was decided that the records of more recent inmates would not be inspected. Other sources were used to investigate and generalize about contemporary patients, notably published studies as well as interviews with hospital personnel.

Around 1960, the methods of keeping records changed. The notations were no longer kept in large books, and the numerical system was abandoned. Now the information was placed in file folders arranged alphabetically using the last name of the patient.

2. E. A. Nahim, *The Drug Problem in Sierra Leone* (Unpublished report, Kissy Mental Hospital, n.d.).

3. O. I. Ifabumuyi, "Alcoholism and Drug Addiction in Northern Nigeria," *Acta Psychiatrica Scandinavica* 73 (1986): 479-80; Adego E. Eferakeya, "Drugs and Suicide Attempts in Benin City, Nigeria," *British Journal of Psychiatry* 145 (1984): 70-73; D. M. Ndetei, P. Kiptong, and K. Odhiambo, "Feighner's Syndrome Profile of Alcoholism in a Kenyan General Hospital," *Acta Psychiatrica Scandinavica* 69 (1984): 409-15; L. Jacobsson, "Acts of Violence in a Traditional Western Ethiopian Society in Transition," *Acta Psychiatrica Scandinavica* 72 (1985): 601-7.

4. Charles R. Swift and Tolani Asuni, *Mental Health and Disease in Africa: With Special Reference to Africa South of the Sahara* (Edinburgh: Churchill Livingstone, 1975), 128-43; G. Allen German, "Aspects of Clinical Psychiatry in Sub-Saharan Africa," *British Journal of Psychiatry* 121 (1972): 461-79; T. Adeoye Lambo, "Neuropsychiatric Observations in the Western Regions of Nigeria," *British Medical Journal* 2 (1956): 1388-94; Lambo, "Further Neuropsychiatric Observations in Nigeria," *British Medical Journal* 11 (1960): 1696-1704.

5. SLA, CR number 4241 (1934-38).

6. H.N.K. arap Mengech and M. Dhadphale, "Attempted Suicide (parasuicide) in Nairobi," *Acta Psychiatrica Scandinavica* 69 (1984): 416-19; L. Jacobsson, "Suicide and Attempted Suicide in a General Hospital in Western Ethiopia, " *Acta Psychiatrica Scandinavica* 71 (1985): 596-600; T. Asuni, "Suicide in Western Nigeria," *British Medical Journal* 3 (1962): 1091-96; S. G. Bloomberg, "The Present State of Suicide Prevention: An African Survey," *International Journal of Social Psychiatry* 128 (1972): 998-1002.

7. T. Duncan Greenlees, "Insanity Among the Natives of South Africa," *Journal of Mental Science* 41 (1895): 71-82; J. C. Carothers, "A Study of Mental Derangement in Africans, and an Attempt to Explain Its Peculiarities, More Especially in Relation to the African Attitude to Life," *Journal of Mental Science* 93 (1947): 47-86; Geoffrey Tooth, *Studies in Mental Illness in the Gold Coast* (London: His Majesty's Stationery Office, 1950).

8. Ayo Binitie, "A Factor-Analytical Study of Depression Across Cultures (African and European)," *British Journal of Psychiatry* 127 (1975): 559.

9. T. Asuni, ed., *Recognition of Depression in the African* (proceedings of the fourth Pan African Congress on Psychiatry, July 1975, Abidjan, Ivory Coast); Raymond Prince, "The Changing Picture of Depressive Syndromes in Africa," *Canadian Journal of African Studies* 1 (1968): 177-92; T. Buchan, "Depression in African Patients," *South African Medical Journal* 43 (1969): 1055-58; O. I. Ifabumuyi, "Demographic Characteristics of Depressives in Northern Nigeria," *Acta Psychiatrica Scandinavica* 68 (1983): 271-76; D. M. Ndetei and A. Vadher, "Types of Life Events Associated with Depression in a Kenyan Setting," *Acta Psychiatrica Scandinavica* 66 (1982): 163-68; D. M. Ndetei and A. Vadher, "Life Events Occurring Before and After Onset of Depression in a Kenyan Setting - Any Significance?" *Acta Psychiatrica Scandinavica* 69 (1984): 327-32; A. Vadher and D. M. Ndetei, "Life Events and Depression in a Kenyan Setting," *British Journal of Psychiatry* 139 (1981): 134-

37; U. H. Ihezue and N. Kumaraswamy, "Socio-Demographic Factors of Depressive Illness Among Nigerians," *Acta Psychiatrica Scandinavica* 73 (1986): 128-32.

10. Ayo Binitie, "A Factor-Analytical Study," 559-63.

11. Ayo Binitie, "The Differentiation of Masked Depression from Psychoneurotic Disorders," in T. Asuni, *Recognition of Depression in the African.* 31-33.

12. Asuni, *Recognition of Depression in the African*, 17-18.

13. Wolfgang G. Jilek and Louise Jilek-Aall, "Transient Psychoses in Africans," *Psychiatrica Clinica* 3 (1970): 337-38.

14. Ibid., 338-64.

6 Hospital and Traditional Care

The care of patients at Kissy Mental Hospital, until quite recent times, has been largely custodial. This is similar to the situation in public mental institutions in other parts of Africa and the world. Beginning in the mid-twentieth century, new therapeutics, chiefly electroconvulsive methods and psychopharmacological treatments, were introduced, and achieved some success. Administrative reforms made the institution more efficient and cost-effective and, most important, restricted the indiscriminate admission of clients. Criminal patients, particularly, could no longer be automatically sent to the facility.

Such gains were important. Yet psychiatric hospital care in Sierra Leone still faces formidable difficulties. It has never been adequately financed; it has never been an issue of national concern, a priority matter demanding swift political resolution. An additional, most restrictive element hampering the growth and development of psychiatry has been the appeal and strength of traditional medicine. This system has been, and remains, a potent and effective rival to modern psychiatry. In a way, the hospital has been an adjunct to the practice of traditional healers.

Historically, the healers have received journalistic and scholarly attention, but much of that literature has attributed negative qualities to indigenous care. Over time, this unfavorable evaluation has been softened, and most contemporary observers view traditional healers as positive contributors to mental health care in developing nations. While conflicts do continue to exist throughout the Third World between traditional medicine and the biomedical system, in Sierra Leone confrontation has been minimal. During the 1980s, for example, the Kissy hospital adminis-

tration cooperated and consulted with numerous traditional practitioners. The hospital leadership recognized the appeal and the
breadth of traditional medicine as well as its powerful
psychotherapeutic impact on clients.

HOSPITAL CARE AND TREATMENT

Throughout the early colonial era, and well into the opening
decades of the twentieth century, the care and treatment at Kissy
hospital aimed at improving and maintaining the physical health
of the inmates. This policy reflected the basically custodial nature
of the institution; it was also a reaction to the large numbers of
patients arriving in a weak, debilitated condition, suffering from
some bodily injury, handicap, or disease. Moreover, many
physicians believed insanity to be a physical condition, so that it
was appropriate to build up the general health of the patient to
help fight the mental disease. The restoration and maintenance of
the inmates' physical health remained a major activity of the hospital.

As observed earlier, varied kinds of medications were prescribed: a ferri tonic was given to the anemic and those persons
weakened by nutritional deficiency. Potassium bromide was used
as a sedative. For a dying patient, sinking fast, strychnine was in-
jected to stimulate the central nervous system. While alba, a laxa-
tive, was administered to relieve constipation; calomel and bis-
muth were purgatives, combatting parasites and diarrhea; and
quinine was utilized to control fever. For about ten years,
through the mid- and late 1930s and into the 1940s, the Kahn
blood test, to detect syphilis, was given to each new patient.

All of these medical measures did enhance the physical well-
being of the inmates. Very few therapies, however, were available that were designed specifically for the care and treatment of
psychiatrically impaired persons. Various tasks and recreational
activities kept some patients preoccupied. Recalcitrant or incorrigible clients were restrained in a modified straitjacket, called
a coverlette, and placed in a special isolation cell.[1]

Beginning in the late-colonial era, notably in the 1950s, and
continuing to the present, the hospital assumed and promoted a
therapeutic role. The institution did remain a custodial facility, a
welfare agency, and a depository for the unruly and unwanted;
these functions were, of course, still common to public mental
hospitals throughout the world. Notwithstanding such burdens,

the administration kept abreast of the latest developments in psychiatric care employed in Western Europe and North America. It supported an outpatient psychiatric clinic at Connaught Hospital, the country's most important medical facility. It encouraged some art, recreational, and occupational therapies. And the two most prominent therapeutics of recent administrative psychiatry, electroconvulsive therapy and psychopharmacological treatment, were applied widely at Kissy.

In American and European mental hospital practice, the use of electric shock therapy faded away quickly in the late 1950s when drugs were introduced for treating the mentally disturbed. Throughout Africa, however, the employment of ECT prevailed into the 1970s. A report from the psychiatric hospital at Enugu, Nigeria, pointed to its efficacy. Here, the practitioners referred to ECT as a "lifesaving treatment" and called for its use at community psychiatric centers. Since the majority of Nigeria's population lived in rural areas, electroconvulsive treatment, its advocates contended, would offer the quickest and best relief to the many psychotics residing in all regions of the country. Along with this general view, the observers at Enugu held that ECT was the most effective with patients suffering from depression, schizophrenia, mania, and puerperal psychosis. It reduced the length of hospitalization for many clients, and some of the more psychotic and violent patients responded well to it.[2]

At Kissy hospital in the early 1960s, electroconvulsive therapy was administered to a variety of psychotics. Most were suffering from schizophrenia or mania; some were depressives, and others were unclassified clients. Results were mixed. As in mental hospitals across the world, at Kissy, treatment remained empirical. That is, the patient's response determined the course and extent of the therapy. One client, a Krio man, was "very frightened of ECT"; after a few sessions, he showed "little change," and the treatment was discontinued. Other patients "improved" or "settled down" with ECT; another inmate remained "inaccessible in spite of a course of ECT." The terms "much improved" or "is brighter" with ECT were recorded frequently on patient records.[3]

Along with the utilization of ECT, a more common practice, emerging in the late 1960s and early 1970s, involved the use of drugs in conjunction with electroconvulsive methods. For example, a manic depressive married woman with three previous hospital admissions was given a session of ECT; she "made a complete recovery" and was sent home and back to her job under a regimen of antidepressant drugs and tanquillizers. For another

patient, ECT brought no change of behavior, while the administration of largactil "produced slight improvement"; after taking
stelazine and artane, however, this client was released on parole.
And a young male inmate improved with ECT and was discharged to the care of his mother. Stelazine was prescribed for
him as maintenance therapy.[4]

By the 1980s, electroconvulsive therapy was used less frequently, and nearly every patient in the hospital was on some type of
antipsychotic medication. Largactil or chlorpromazine, mellaril,
and stelazine were dispensed regularly in the wards. Varied
antidepressants were also used. The anticonvulsant phenobar-
bitane was employed commonly to control patients with epilepsy.
Geriatric and poorly nourished clients received large quantities of
vitamin tablets. In effect, a total drug regimen operated at Kissy
hospital, an administrative program common to mental institutions in other African and Western countries.

The results of this approach corresponded to the generally favorable impact of drug treatments on patients and psychiatric
agencies throughout the world. The acceptance and wide applications of psychopharmaceutical therapy facilitated an open and
positive institutional atmosphere. Patients were quiet and
pacified; staff no longer remained on the defensive, functioning
as guards, anticipating trouble and abuse. The need for restraints
and seclusion rooms lessened. Drug therapy, in short, calmed
patients and staff, generating hope and providing relief from the
tedium and noise of institutional life. And more clients, under
prescribed medication with outpatient status, were released into
the community.

Beginning in the 1980s, and concurrent with the psychotropic
drug program, the hospital administration initiated a major policy
change regarding admissions and discharges. Some of the more
formal procedures were dropped. A certificate of emergency was
no longer needed for the hospitalization of a client. Voluntary admissions were encouraged. Relatives or friends might accompany
a person to Kissy for psychiatric examination.

An important new requirement was the acceptance of a contract, a mutually approved arrangement, between the hospital and
the client's relatives. The contract specified that the incoming
patient would not remain institutionalized for more than three
months. This policy militated against overcrowding, and it frustrated any attempt to incarcerate an unwanted relative for a long
period of time. The hospital administration also stopped the influx of large numbers of the criminally insane. Prisoners suffer-

ing from real or apparent mental illness were observed and treated at a psychiatric unit located in the main prison in Freetown.[5]

This effort at limiting the direct flow of criminals to Kissy from prisons throughout the country did not change a basic pattern of patient referral to the hospital. The police continued to bring in a significant number of clients: these individuals had committed an act of violence or engaged in foolish or threatening behavior, becoming a nuisance or danger to the community.

This general condition of behavior of incoming patients constituted a major feature of the Kissy clientele. It can be verified clearly by examining the reasons given for admission on patient records. An analysis of the case notes of a sample of 512 patients over the 1960s and early 1970s indicates that 305 were sent to the mental hospital because of violent activities.[6]

Some of these persons were designated simply "violent and aggressive." One man had "a history of violence"; he was "very uncooperative and hostile." Another individual was "restless and violent, attacking innocent people with sticks and a machete." A male paranoid schizophrenic "chased people with a cutlass." A woman heard voices, "asking her to do bad things," and she assaulted people in her household. Another man was "violent to his wife"; he attacked people in the streets and destroyed property at home. A woman "suddenly turned psychotic" and became violent.

In several instances, people were caught in embarrassing and undignified situations as well as threatening violent behavior. One individual was described as "violent, boisterous," a man who "roams the streets always in the nude." Another man was "found in the middle of the road, raving, indecently dressed." A woman "shouts insults and enters residences naked." Another female was "standing and lying in the highway, obstructing traffic." One middle-aged woman "roams streets talking to herself" and became "violent at times."

While many of these persons were criminal offenders, many were also in desperate need of psychiatric care. They were generally schizophrenic and delusional, suffering from some acute psychotic disorder or drug and alcohol dependency. In many of the cases, the patient was hospitalized for safekeeping, detention, and isolation, with only incidental concern for treatment and care. This situation diminished the therapeutic role of the institution, and reflected the fact that the hospital at Kissy was recognized by the populace as a custodial facility. For the majority of patients, incarceration represented a last resort, a way out of a difficult situation. The institution was the place to go when familial and other sources of support were drained and when native or traditional modes of treatment were exhausted.

TRADITIONAL MEDICINE: ISSUES AND CONTROVERSY

In Sierra Leone, and throughout Africa, the traditional healer has played a major role in providing mental health care. Over the years, colonial and Western observers have attached to this person such labels as witch doctor, medicine man, and shaman. Each designation connoted a measure of disdain and ridicule, identifying an individual who allegedly engaged in bizarre and irrational behavior. Indeed, the medicine man frequently had psychopathic qualities attributed to him: he suffered from fear neurosis or hysteria or some personality disorder, and hovered on the edge of insanity. Throughout the early twentieth century, prevailing anthropological opinion characterized him as a psychiatrically disturbed individual.

In the literature of more recent years, this view of the medicine man as a socio- or psychopath has been challenged.[7] Now this person is called a traditional healer and has gained respect and praise. Reports laud his or her efforts: among the Shona in Zimbabwe, he or she practices "an art with superb skill"; in Ghana, the healer is "frequently a psychotherapist of no mean order"; and Yoruba native doctors in Nigeria have "considerable skill and competence in handling psychotherapeutic problems."[8] Other more general reports note that African healers "approach their clients with consideration, warmth, and sympathy."[9] And an empirical study of the effectiveness of a Nigerian herbalist treatment program revealed that six months after discharge, one client was readmitted and 25 percent of the group remained severely ill; all the other patients seemed recovered and completely normal.[10] Such recent evidence undercuts the earlier anthropological representations of witch doctors as psychopaths. Contemporary findings portray traditional healers as effective psychotherapists in their own communities.

At present, a large segment of African and Western opinion calls for the utilization of traditional healers to help resolve the problems of mental health care throughout Africa. A notable step in this direction occurred at Aro, near Abeokuta, Nigeria, under the direction of the Nigerian psychiatrist T. Adeoye Lambo. Starting in 1954, the Aro project, an experiment in community mental health, fused the milieu of a psychiatric day hospital with communal living in nearby villages. In effect, the patients received Western-type treatment in the hospital and traditional care in the villages.

The hospital, a two-hundred bed facility, could offer electroconvulsive therapy and insulin treatments as well as psychopharmacological medication. Usually the patients received various therapies at the institution and returned to their villages late in the afternoon. Here a family member took care of the client, attending to such domestic chores as making meals, washing clothes, and escorting the patient to and from the hospital. The daily regimen involved traditional healers who provided care and social services to clients and collaborated with the hospital staff. No one was isolated in a strange and disturbing place. The center of the patient's life remained in the village, a setting that fostered and encouraged social bonding with family, friends, and community leaders.

Lambo argued that this kind of social matrix greatly enhanced a client's recovery; it kept a patient amidst healthy persons, permitting spontaneous group interactions in a tolerant milieu similar to a patient's home community. In short, by duplicating the basic African social order, the small village, traditional roles and group experiences were exploited as the major therapeutic tools for healing patients.[11]

The efforts of Lambo and other African psychiatrists at integrating indigenous and scientific modes of treatment reflect a basic reality of African mental health care: traditional healers provide services valued by their clients. This is not disputed. It is recognized that traditional doctors specialize largely in treating the psychiatrically impaired. They handle more cases of mental disorder than any other kind of illness. Several factors encourage the mentally distraught to seek their help. The local healer is a familiar member of the community, well-known to the patient and his kin group. To the client, the healer's proximity and sociability make him or her a dependable, acceptable person who can offer help and solace.

Also, throughout Africa, only a few persons trained in modern psychiatry and psychology are available to consumers; on the other hand, there are large numbers of traditional healers, providing all sorts of options to the public. Most significant, the majority of clients, kin, and healers share similar views regarding the etiology and cure of mental illness. There is a commonality of beliefs, values, and symbols. Madness is attributed to the influence of mystical or supernatural forces, sometimes called witchcraft, invoked, most likely, by an unfriendly person or party. This belief is pervasive and frustrates the practitioners of modern psychiatry. The traditional healer, however, recognizes the social reality of supernatural causation; he or she shares the psychological world of the client, and devises ways for the client to overcome the fears and anxieties engendered by unseen and malevolent forces.

Of special significance is the integration of the mentally ill person into various group rituals and processes of healing. During the stages of treatment, in other words, the traditional healer involves family members, tapping powerful ties of support and affect between client and kin. As a family and community observer, the healer can offer meaningful social explanations for illness. All of the shared experiences in curing the client, in reintegrating him or her back into the community, facilitates the genial acceptance of the indigenous practitioner. Viewing this person as a mentor, client and kin accept his or her methods and advice, and carry out instructions and prescriptions without fear or dread of the consequences. This trust is reciprocated by the healer, who recognizes the family as the manager of the mentally ill relative. The family, not the individual client, consults and deals with the practitioner, establishing a brokerage and therapeutic arrangement that prevails until the patient returns to the community.[12]

Studies of the clientele of traditional healers in African cities have presented some generally uniform findings. Patients and kin groups shop around for native doctors, and more treatment choices are available to city residents than to people living in the country. Throughout rural Africa, indigenous health care remains the basic, and, in many places, the only available medical system. Some religious institutions offer support services in both village and city environments. In urban settings, however, modern medicine has a historical and institutional base, and competes with traditional medicine for patients. While most of the clients of urban healers represent new cases, a significant number are former patients, or have received care from other indigenous doctors.

Aside from this feature, reports on client characteristics point to the importance of two variables: gender and education. Women utilize the services of native healers more than men.

Many of the complaints relate to reproductive matters, called "womb trouble," including barrenness, repeated miscarriages, and disturbed pregnancies. Women also seek out healers for support in resolving marital and family problems as well as stresses in the workplace. Petty marketing, the ubiquitous activity of African women, brings uncertainties and failures, lending itself to personalistic, supernatural explanations for misfortune. In such circumstances, a traditional healer might offer solace and protection.

The findings of a study of thirty traditional doctors located in Abeokuta, Nigeria, ran counter to prevailing professional opinion, indicating the predominance of male clients. The existence of local maternity clinics offered an explanation. Here women and children received treatment, utilizing a service different from traditional medicine.

While most reports show more women than men using traditional care, another variable, educational status, may determine the attitude toward, and the degree of acceptance of, indigenous healers. A research project in southern Nigeria involving 150 subjects - 75 university students and 75 market traders with a lower level of education - revealed generally negative opinions about mental illness. All believed that a mentally ill relative should remain a family matter, a secret to be kept from the wider community.

Opinions differed over etiology and respect for healers. The market people accepted traditional views on the cause of mental illness; the students were more skeptical about attributing mental disorder to the machinations of hostile persons or forces. The market traders feared native healers more than the students did, and they also believed, in contrast to the university group, that Western trained physicians knew little about treating mental illness.

Other studies have confirmed these findings, demonstrating that persons with a higher education tend to disregard native medicine. Still, the view of the majority of the people, as presented in recent research, places less importance on education, and affirms respect for native healers who, it is believed, have the therapeutic skills needed to combat and cure mentally disordered persons. One pattern is clear and obvious: clients look around. When options exist, they commute between traditional and modern medical personnel and institutions. In numerous instances, clients obtain treatment simultaneously from psychologists or psychiatrists at clinics or hospitals, and from traditional doctors.[13]

Several types of traditional healers have prevailed throughout Africa. The categories vary with the region and the ethnic group, and, at times, their functions and identities merge and overlap. The herbalist has remained the most prominent and respected kind of traditional practitioner. After a long period of apprenticeship, the herbalist acquires an empirical, naturalistic orientation. This healer relies on herbal medicine, treating illness or adversity by means of herbs, roots, and barks. A client inhales the vapors of a boiling mixture, sits in a brew, or drinks it, or has it rubbed on his body.

While some magico-religious techniques, such as incantations and sacrifices, are employed, the herbalist does not engage in harmful practices directed at others. He might indulge in defensive or protective magic, and prepare a talisman. Many herbalists receive patients at their houses on specific days and hours of the week. Others sell herbal ingredients and animal materials such as skins, feathers, and bones at markets; some distribute patent medicines and Western drugs.

The diviner, or diviner-priest or -priestess, is another type of traditional practitioner. Herbalists and diviners often use similar techniques and methods. Some herbalists learn the arts of divination, many diviners are skilled in herbal medicine. The diviner, through an oracle divinity, or bone divination, diagnoses a problem - a condition of bad health or misfortune - and prescribes a course of action - most often a ritual and animal sacrifice. The shrine priest also conducts sacrifices, as well as rituals of appeasement and thanksgiving.

On the other hand, the sorcerer healer offers a cure to a disorder, but can also cause an illness. He elicits fear and mistrust by his willingness to exploit his knowledge, skills, and magic towards harmful ends. The magician healer's charm, an amulet or fetish, checks the threat of the sorcerer. Worn around the neck or waist, the charm consists usually of a braided or knotted string of different colors. During its preparation, incantations, which give the client protection, are pronounced over the charm. This guardian spirit presumably resides in the knot forever. In Muslim areas, the marabout, or alpha man, carries considerable prestige and authority to deal with mental patients. He too employs charms, ritual and written, for preventing and treating illness.

There are other names for traditional practitioners. A native doctor is tagged a curative, or a psychic, or a spiritual healer. On occasion, the designations medicine man and witch doctor are used; and everywhere African terms are applied. Generally, a traditional healer takes an eclectic approach, utilizing and borrowing assorted techniques and practices, some unique to a locality and other methods widespread throughout the continent.

In sum, two features characterize the African healer: a reliance on herbal medicine which the practitioner prepares by hand, and an acceptance of a world view that interprets mental illness as a supernatural, antisocial phenomenon, a disorder that can be treated and cured by means of integrative group rituals and experiences as well as herbal remedies.[14]

Conflict and controversy have agitated the relationship between traditional medicine and the biomedical system. Since the 1970s, an assortment of interests and groups have called for collaboration between indigenous practitioners and modern medical personnel. This diverse coalition includes international health agencies, governments eager to cut costs, nationalists determined to develop a national medical system, pharmacologists seeking new drugs, psychiatrists sensitive to resolving patient problems in other cultures, critics of drug companies and of the claims of Western medicine, Western anthropologists, public health officials, and assorted scholars. Despite the rhetoric, the interest, and the support, few programs of collaboration exist.

Several factors militate against cooperation. The cultural differences between the two systems may be too wide to bridge. The modern physician has difficulty understanding and appreciating the beliefs of the traditional healer. This alienation can turn to professional envy or suspicion if an urban indigenous practitioner has a lucrative practice that takes patients away from the physician.

Reports of abuse and malpractice damage the status and authority of traditional healers. Some practitioners flog clients routinely, believing that by doing so they are driving evil spirits away. Patients have arrived at hospitals with bruises and marks left by whips, and wounds on ankles and wrists caused by being shackled in chains. Critics point to examples of bad practices: a healer in Swaziland gave herbal enemas to children with infectious diarrhea; a marabout in Mali wrote Koranic charms on the backs of patients suffering from cholera. Concern has been also expressed over the use of potent psychotropic herbs such as rauwolfia, without apparent accurate measurement of doses or control over and sensitivity to the side effects of this powerful medication.

While such reports may be biased and based on the information of disgruntled and dissatisfied clients, they do point to a major problem. The open, fluid, and varied nature of traditional medicine allows charlatans and opportunists to profit. They can exploit popular beliefs and promise a cure for any kind of illness. Traditional healers are not monitored by any agency; they are neither regulated nor subjected to censure. They engage in diverse practices based on different levels and standards of training and knowledge.

This situation persists, and frustrates efforts at incorporating healers into a national health system. Some government officials also maintain that indigenous practitioners represent an anachronism, a throwback to a primitive, backward time, and, that they stand in the way of progress, of building a modern nation. In Marxist societies, such as Mozambique and Tanzania, traditional healers are viewed with mild disdain, as figures of the past, of an unproductive, superstitious feudal order.[15]

The argument that traditional healers contribute little to a modern medical system is diminished by the reality of health care in most African societies. A shortage of trained personnel exists everywhere. With such widespread resource deficiencies, traditional healers help fill the gap. Political and medical policy makers recognize that a nation's health goals cannot be achieved without indigenous practitioners. Also, traditional medicine offers a unique contribution: it fills a social and personal need, especially where the biomedical system is most vulnerable, namely, in the delivery of mental health care.

Clients and traditional physicians know the strengths of scientific medicine: it has effective immunization programs; it has brought relief to such epidemic diseases as yaws and sleeping sickness; it provides excellent care in pediatrics, gynecology and surgery. In most instances, indigenous practitioners do not enter such areas of biomedical competence.

Psychiatry, however, seems an imprecise and uncertain field; its clients recover slowly and by means of an invisible process. Here, traditional healers can compete effectively. Sensitive to the social dimensions of illness as well as popular beliefs, traditional healers answer the demands of clients. Accessible and credible, they help people coping with the psychosomatic effects of failure, unemployment, witchcraft, and magic, along with the misunderstandings arising from social and family conflict, realms of life largely outside the range of Western medicine. Significantly, the therapy of native practitioners always succeeds in at least one sense: the healers reassure clients and relieve anxieties. Popular confidence in them remains high, even if they cannot cure an affliction or remove the symptoms.[16]

Recent literature extols the virtues of collaboration between traditional medicine and the biomedical system.[17] Some traditional healers in urban areas seem willing to adapt and cooperate with modern medical personnel. They may employ the outward trappings of Western-trained physicians. For example, they may have wheelchairs, use a stethoscope and a thermometer when examining a patient, utilize bandages, and, if possible, Xrays. Some collaborate with health officials. This arrangement brings them social and economic benefits, notably, an expanded practice and an opportunity to sell commodities promoted by government authorities and foreign firms.

However, at least through the 1980s, widespread cooperation between the two medical systems has been a stated future national goal rather than an actual day-to-day reality. In both camps, suspicions abound. Healers fear absorption and domination by political authorities determined to modernize health care. Psychiatrists do respect the psychotherapeutic contributions of healers, but remain wary of charlatans and the lack of quality control over the activities of traditional practitioners.

Further, throughout the continent, psychiatric illness is not recognized as a pressing public health problem. The limited medical and financial resources of African countries force them to focus on such major concerns as malnutrition, infectious disease, and parasitic infestations. This reality alone dictates that traditional approaches to mental health care will prevail for a long time.

TRADITIONAL MEDICINE AND INSANITY IN RURAL SIERRA LEONE

Traditional medicine in Sierra Leone represents a microcosm of African indigenous mental health care. Here, and across sub-Saharan Africa, a general etiological assumption provides the basic rationale for traditional treatment: a powerful and widespread belief in the supernatural causation of madness maintains and facilitates the growth of the system of indigenous medicine and practitioners. Biomedical authorities at Kissy Mental Hospital observe that people throughout the country view mental illness as a great stigma - indeed, a curse, a manifestation of evil. It is not seen as a disease or a behavioral disorder. The sufferer may be a victim of someone's wrath or envy. Also, the sick person, or one of the patient's relatives, may have committed some social or personal offense, and so the client's distraught mental condition represents a form of punishment. This pervasive system of belief accounts in large part for the popularity of traditional practitioners: they tell people the source of illness and can deal effectively with its mystical causes.[18]

The violation of a community norm affects profoundly an individual's life and health. Among the Kuranko in eastern Sierra Leone, a person's failure to honor or show respect for one's ancestors may have a fatal result. For example, after two young Kuranko men had been killed in a lorry accident far away from their homes, a village elder in Kuranko country noted that the two men had cut themselves off from their communities. They had repudiated the past, rejecting a traditional life-style, and sought work as wage laborers. This action brought their destruction, the elder claimed. By ignoring their responsibilities, notably by neglecting to offer sacrifices to dead relatives and by rebuffing the elders, the young men lost the protection of ancestor spirits and became vulnerable to the insecurities of an alien world.[19]

While this event had an unfortunate ending, more typically a Kuranko consults a healer or a diviner when faced with a social crisis or change. After a consultation, a sacrifice of raw rice flour is offered and a ritual performed to avert disorder and maintain social harmony.[20] A neighboring people of the Kuranko, the Kono, engage in a similar ritual when confronted with an unexplained illness. The diviner determines the cause of the sickness, and might conclude that the client has stolen something or offended an elderly relative. Whatever the cause, the diviner, the client, and his family gather for a ceremony of confession and offerings. The client admits guilt, is forgiven, and gifts are presented. After some herbal medicine is prescribed and reassuring words spoken, the ceremony ends with the participants eating rice.[21]

Along with other ethnic groups in Sierra Leone, the Kuranko place high value on good health. To them, a healthy person is physically strong and well built, has a hearty appetite, and is happy and free of worry. Some of the essentials for assuring health include an adequate and wholesome diet, well-cooked food, cleanliness in the preparation of meals, and uncontaminated water. A community may select its water supply and everyone must take responsibility to ensure its purity.

When sickness occurs, a herbalist will most likely be sought to prepare medicine from roots, barks, and herbs, and to prescribe diet restrictions to clients. Here again the healer may be asked to resolve a patient's transgression or infringement on some personal or community taboo. For example, the Kuranko believe that a man will become ill if he spies on women at their special sanctuary, a place designated by the village where they may bathe privately and attend to personal matters. Illness will also result if a person spies on the activities of a secret society of the opposite sex. And serious illness will follow if one party violates an agreement made between two closely related persons. In each of these instances, by means of confession and ritual cleansings, the healer will mediate the disruption, assure social peace, and cure the client.[22]

Above all, the Kuranko fear uncontrollable, external supernatural forces that can harm one's health and in some cases destroy life itself. These may include witches, sorcerers, bush spirits or human enemies. The forces may be contained and neutralized by means of an assortment of charms, fetishes, and medicines. Acquired from a healer, or mori-man, such defenses may include a padlock wrapped with white, red, and black threads, which allegedly has the power to immobilize a victim. Another device consists of a cord with a noose. It is supposed to have the force to bind a person mystically. It takes effect when a few words are spoken, the victim's name mentioned, and the noose is jerked tightly around a clenched fist. A different cord, specified for stopping evil from entering a house, is made of twisted white and black threads and is hung over the threshold of a room. Other types of defenses might include a liquid medicine that is rubbed on the body, or a charm worn around the neck.[23] All of these devices constitute precautionary measures, or preventive medicine, designed to combat and control the unpredictable and unseen forces of envy and evil.

This pattern of defense is followed by other groups throughout the country, including the Susu and the Limba, peoples occupying areas west of the Kuranko. Each one recognizes the importance of ancestral spirits in directing the lives of people. Sacrifices, prayers, and incantations show respect for elders and keep the dead spirits alert to the social events of the village. Negligence in the performance of such duties might result in sickness. Each ethnic group senses the power of witchcraft to threaten and harm one's health and well-being. Varied measures are taken to prevent and detect it. Men, women, and children wear amulets and charms. Like the Kuranko, the Limba hang protective devices, such as pieces of leather, native cloth, wicker, and perhaps a dead spider, over the doorways of huts.[24]

A common practice, particularly in the hinterland, is invoking a "swear," or a curse, a publicly approved and controlled event aimed at a malefactor, rival, or enemy. It is directed often against some offender, such as a thief. Before a swear is formally pronounced, the permission of the village chief is obtained and the owner of the stolen article makes a threat that is broadcast throughout the community, asking the wrongdoer to come forward and admit guilt. If no confession occurs, the next morning a swear is proclaimed, asserting that the guilty person will be caught and suffer a terrible punishment.

The punishment might occur in a few weeks, or it could happen some years after the declaration of the swear. In any event, it is taken most seriously and is greatly feared. The prevailing assumption is that a swear may kill someone or make a person sick, crazy, or impotent. When illness does occur, the swear is always a possible cause.[25] Worry over a curse may cause an individual to succumb to extreme anxiety and dread, and the person may appear psychologically abnormal. Relief from this situation of stress and strain comes with a confession, which releases the curse and, at the same time, reintegrates the individual into the community.[26]

Secret societies also play a role in controlling aberrant behavior. The Poro of the Temne, Mende, and Sherbro, and for the women, the Bundo or Sande, offer guidelines of conduct that orient individuals and assure group identity and solidarity. Medical practices and the treatment of the sick are functions of secret societies. The elder members are the specialists and practitioners who can manipulate magical and mystical power, giving them immense prestige and power in the community. Their role, and indeed the major purpose of the society, is laying down the law, determining conduct and behavior. It is believed that a breach of a rule or regulation places an individual in danger of becoming ill.

Among the Mende, insanity results from some transgression of the Njayei society. The sufferer may have trespassed on the territory of the association or seen the dead body of an important Njayei official before it was purified. In such instances, initiation into the society is the apparent cure for the sickness. The individual is not alone; his sickness affects all the people tied closely to him, and they must share responsibility for the breach of conduct as well as be a part of the treatment process. The initiation and purification rituals will release anxiety, expiate the guilt, externalize responsibility, and reintegrate the sick person and his relatives into the community.[27] All of this confirms the group approach to African medical and psychiatric practice, a contrast to the individualism of the developed world, where care focuses largely on a doctor-patient relationship.

URBAN SOCIAL DISORDER AND ANOMIE

In urban areas of Sierra Leone, namely Freetown, traditional secret societies of the provinces such as the Poro have had less influence and control and have been supplanted by various voluntary organizations. Some relate to the early-nineteenth-century Freetown associations of the Aku, the liberated slaves of Yoruba origin. In confronting sickness and death, this ethnic group sought comfort and help by means of a traditional practice: Gelede masked dancers performed to entertain and appease witches, the presumed source of sickness. A sacrifice of a sheep would be followed by a ritual involving its blood mixed with palm oil; people dipped their hands in this mixture to ward off a disease. The cult of the Shango and the ancestral Egungun cult also sought a cure for sickness, as well as safety from witches, by making sacrifices and dancing as masqueraders in the streets. A more restrained way of contacting and receiving the blessings of ancestral spirits was the Krio ritual feast, of Yourba origin, called the awujoh. It took place after the birth of a child, or before a marriage. If some misfortune occurred, an awujoh was held to gain forgiveness from angered spirits, who, it was believed, had caused the adversity.[28]

Outside the Krio community, other kinds of associations evolved as more ethnic groups from the protectorate migrated to Freetown around 1900. These arrivals, chiefly young men, were not easily assimilated into the city's existing population. Illiterate and unskilled, with little facility in English or Krio, they remained separate and under their own leaders.

The colonial government recognized this situation, and it created and fostered a system of tribal authorities. Under this program, a tribal ruler or headman administered to the needs of his ethnic group in Freetown. Officially inaugurated in 1905 as "An Ordinance to Promote a System of Administration by Tribal Authority Among the Tribes Settled in Freetown," by the time of the outbreak of World War I, tribal rulers were recognized for seven ethnic groups. The most important included the Temne, Mende, Limba, and Kroo.[29]

Over time, the headman and his retinue offered an array of basic services to newly arrived migrants. These might include securing temporary housing, finding jobs, arranging burial services, paying bail for arrested persons, and mediating conflicts of individuals within the group and with other people. The settlement of domestic disputes in courtlike settings proved a most acceptable arrangement for the group. Here the headman resolved matters that were largely outside the concern and purview of government authorities.[30]

Many of the problems dealt with witchcraft. One headman heard complaints about a person with a witchgun who, it was claimed, brought sickness to his neighbors. Other cases involved threats to the health and safety of children. In one instance, a child died after a long illness. This fact, however, was not accepted by the grieving parents, who charged eight persons with casting bad medicine on the infant, causing its death. In another case, several women exchanged witchcraft accusations, and death threats were directed at the child of the youngest female of the group. All of this was complicated by a tangle of conflicting evidence and emotions, with the elusive witch remaining undetected. The headman resolved the matter, as he noted, in the "native way," by requiring that each member of the party take out a swear; this curse, he argued, would eventually find and punish the guilty person.

Along with threats to children and charges of sorcery, headmen were preoccupied with marital problems, including men who claimed that the medicine of their wives had made them impotent. One man went further and blamed his spouse for ruining his life. The trouble started when the wife, unable to conceive a child, went to an alpha man for advice and medicine. After both the husband and wife drank the healer's mixtures, they quarreled violently and he ordered her out of the house. The matter, however, did not end there. The medicine, the husband claimed, continued to effect him adversely; it gave him a negative attitude and he was dismissed from his job. He became ill and spent sums of money on medicines and professional advice.

The headman resolved this dilemma by requiring that the wife pay a small fine; in addition, she would meet with her husband and the alpha man who had prepared the liquid, and another healer would be present who would inform the husband that he had not been ruined by the alpha's medicine.[31]

Voluntary organizations, along with the headmen, gave the migrants material and moral support as well as supernatural protection. These groups proliferated after World War I, as migration from the protectorate to Freetown increased. To a lesser degree, this movement of people seeking opportunity and escape affected the smaller cities of Sierra Leone, namely Bo, Kenema, and Port Loko.

Ambas Geda, meaning bringing together, was a typical association formed in Freetown in the early 1930s to meet the needs of migrants. Its organizers lamented the apparent loss of ethnic identity among Temne youth in the city. Some young people, isolated and remote from home communities and living in a seemingly alien city, succumbed to psychological disturbances. Ambas Geda provided social outlets to its members; its entertainment and welfare activities fostered a group identity, relieving individual anxiety and anomie. In effect, Ambas Geda, and similar associations called compins or companies, offered emotional satisfaction. They kept together persons of like interests and ethnic affiliation.[32]

During and after World War II, large-scale migration to Freetown intensified, and new types of voluntary organizations emerged. Many of these rural migrants, as well as poor indigents of the city, had few social, verbal, or job skills, and became part of a new underclass of the unemployed. Some were involved in gangs, petty crime, and drug abuse.

Such problems, particularly juvenile delinquency, caught the attention of the government. The increasing numbers of young offenders, popularly called wharf rats, elicited official concern and commentary.[33] In February 1941, for example, the Freetown commissioner of police informed the colonial secretary about the growing juvenile population in the prisons and attributed it to his "crusade against wharf rats." On the other hand, he observed that the war had brought to Freetown many European sailors who were "free with their money," a situation that encouraged youngsters to chase after them hoping to pick some easy cash. Parents and teachers complained, the commissioner noted, about their young people running away from school and mingling with the seamen. This contact, it was felt, threatened morals and facilitated juvenile crime.[34]

The colonial government delegated responsibility for supervising and reforming juvenile delinquents in the colony - that is, Freetown and environs - to ministers of various religious denominations. Accordingly, the Reverend A. Stott of the Sierra Leone District Synod of the Methodist Church took the initiative and prepared a substantial analysis of the criminal activities among the young of Freetown. This document, "Report on the Nature and Extent of the Problem of Juvenile Delinquency in

Sierra Leone," made no reference to war or foreign sailors. Instead it pointed to protectorate youth, experiencing "detribalization," as the major source of juvenile offenders in Freetown. These young people were cut off from family, home, and community - the small, safe, self-contained villages of the hinterland. In the city, a strange, artificial, foreign environment, they experienced a "fearful sense of loneliness." Their familial and communal bonds were missing; they had few meaningful activities; they had no work and little chance of finding employment. The city, with its cosmopolitan and mercantile atmosphere, stimulated new needs, desires,and temptations that could not be easily gratified. To find security and indulgence, some youths turned to a life of petty crime.

Stott's report did not present figures demonstrating an alarming increase in the number of juvenile delinquents. Instead, it claimed that most crimes went unrecorded, and most offenders escaped justice; consequently, any statistical study showing a low incidence of crime represented a deception and did not reveal the actual extent of the problem. On the basis of the information in this report, the majority of offenders were illiterate boys between 13 and 15 years of age who had committed some act of petty theft. There were only a few cases of assault and disorderly behavior. Flogging was the chief mode of punishment, an unfortunate fact but, the report continued, the only realistic option because these delinquents had no home or family around which another focus of treatment could be structured and administered. The document concluded with an "urgent" recommendation that a home be provided where juvenile remand and detention cases could be sent. An official notation on this report concurred with that conclusion.[35]

A police magistrate in Freetown also affirmed the need for a place to send delinquents, warning the colonial secretary that government action to control young offenders could not be postponed. He argued that the situation in Freetown resembled conditions in Kingston, Jamaica. In that West Indian city, government inaction and negligence had allowed a social problem to fester and grow and reach the point where it was a daily event for gangs of "young hooligans" to terrorize and rob people and shops in the downtown streets. The police official believed that the conditions for a similar predicament were growing in Freetown: a large influx of people looking for work, increasing unemployment, bad housing conditions, a developing consciousness of exploitation, no playing fields or recreational facilities to keep young people off the streets, and a lack of family and community discipline and restraints. To cope with the problems of youthful offenders, he called upon the government to consider appointing probation officers, creating boys clubs, and establishing a reformatory.[36]

While the government debated the merits of such proposals, youths themselves formed voluntary organizations called Ode-lay societies. These groups were related to the compins of the 1930s as well as the Yoruba Gelede and Egungun traditions of the nineteenth century, and in contemporary Freetown they remain very popular. Their clientele come from the young and largely unemployed. Ode-lay associations give members an identity, a sense of belonging. They offer social interactions, entertainments, music, and, their most dramatic events, masquerades and processions.

All these gatherings, as well as the members themselves are protected by the group's powerful "medicine." The term medicine is misnomer. Juju is the Krio word for medicine; the Freetown Yoruba term is ogun. In a West African context, medicine, or juju or ogun, connotes a worldview, embracing all facets of life. It is rooted in indigenous religion and is a force that can destroy or protect, bring good or bad luck, heal or cause illness. It has a sensitive, private nature and is at the core of any secret society in Freetown, including Ode-lay organizations.

Perhaps the most confidential aspect of these groups is its medicine. While not losing its mysterious, mystical characteristics, the medicine can become a very concrete matter. The initiates of a group, for example, may eat the medicine, the juju. It may be called soweh, which is a concoction of crushed vegetables combined with palm oil or water and animal blood. After taking the soweh, a person dramatically, and intimately, achieves full membership, becoming an organic part of the society. For protection, a participant in a masquerade ceremony may sprinkle the mixture on a costume or rub it on his body.[37] The juju, of course, is not simply a concoction; it goes beyond mere material substance. This ubiquity, particularly its power to control a person or an event, is what captures and holds the imagination of the participants and believers.

URBAN HEALERS

It is within this social milieu of beliefs, an atmosphere of apparently strong and hidden, sometimes malevolent forces that may cause disorder and illness, that traditional healers thrive and prosper. In present-day Freetown, a herbalist magician advertises his skills in a local newspaper, claiming that he has practiced the arts of healing in forty-two countries. While asserting that "a gift of God" made him a doctor, he confesses that his knowledge and training came from his father and mother; both were healers, and he took pride in inheriting this family business.

His place of practice is a residence located just a few blocks from the heart of the city. Here a client is brought into a dark, windowless room. A small bed stands against a wall, and off to the side are assorted bottles and a large pile of cans of condensed milk. The healer, a large middle-aged man with a commanding appearance, sits in a chair behind a small table illuminated only by two large candles. The client and his party sit in chairs opposite the table. Behind the healer, on a shelf high up on the wall, there are several pictures: the details of these representations vary, but each shows a healer with a large snake in the foreground.

While this Freetown healer will not take difficult, violent patients, he recognizes four categories of mental disorder: one kind exhibits epileptic fits, a second may be labeled hypomania and involves running about with a broken bottle, a third is represented by a quiet, depressed person, and a final type results from some accident or brain injury.

This healer's treatment process follows a basic pattern. During the initial evaluation interview, the main consideration of the practitioner is to make the client happy and physically content. He "sprays the air," and the patient takes a short nap. An herb mixed with milk brings refreshment. The client has been told that a snake has returned from the bush with a herb that will give him relief.

Above all, this herbalist magician emphasizes the power of witchcraft to cause pain and suffering. Everyone, he contends, needs protection from the evil spells that witches cast over a person. He relates a case of an African woman who returned home after having a baby in Europe. An evil person, a witch, placed a hex on the baby. The woman went back to Europe, and the infant became sick with fever and chronic pain. European medicines and treatments offered no relief. The woman came home to Africa, consulted a healer - clearly it was this Freetown herbalist magician - and the baby was cured. It was accomplished by rubbing medicine on the practitioner's fingers and then touching the infant.

The story emphasizes the need for protection against evil individuals or forces out to destroy a person. This healer provided ways to ward off the danger. The snake had brought the appropriate herb for the client. Protection is achieved by drinking the herb with milk or rubbing it over the body; it can be mixed with perfume, vaseline, or palm oil.

A charm, or sebe, may also thwart an evil-doer. It consists of a string or thin strip of cloth or leather worn about the waist, neck, wrist, or arm. A secretive and brief ritual, performed by a healer, has given the sebe powerful protective strengths that it presumably never loses. The healer warns that without the sebe a person becomes vulnerable to witchcraft.

In his conversations with the sick person, this practitioner warns continuously about the ubiquity of sorcery. He attributes its pervasiveness to the nature of the African mind as well as to the jealousies and resentments aroused in an underdeveloped society characterized by general poverty. In a community of deprivation, he argues, people envy a successful individual - a businessman, doctor, lawyer, or politician - and will wish that some harm befalls that person.

Sensitive to this apparent danger, and convinced that some evil lurks behind any personal problem, he offers largely protective devices and services. He admits being a "black magic man" who operates a business. All of his clients are outpatients; they come, take his advice and medicine, pay a fee, and leave. The sessions are brief; the clients receive what they need and want and feel apparent relief. The practitioner, too, is satisfied, believing that he has contributed to the well-being of the people.[38]

In Kissy, a Muslim herbalist practices a short distance from the mental hospital. He is in his early fifties, of medium height and slender build, and has a quiet, dignified manner. For a long time, he served as an apprentice to his father, learning the rituals and practices of the healing trade as well as the herb prescriptions. This training and knowledge has remained a family secret, a tradition he traces back to his great-grandfather.

The healer accepts all kinds of patients and has facilities in his compound for housing clients over a limited time period. He meets with a client in a room furnished with a large bed, a small two-drawer dresser, a box table, a large wooden chest, a few cushions and low stools. He kneels before the client and family when conducting the therapy sessions.

During the treatment process, the healer may utilize the liquids contained in six glass flasks standing on top of the chest. Each of these herb mixtures has a special function. The type and quantity to be administered is determined by the client's behavior and physical condition. The liquid from one bottle pacifies a wild and intractable patient. It is sprayed in the air around the sick person. The healer claims that the vapors and fumes quiet an unruly individual. In conjunction with this measure, a portion of the contents from a second flask is taken by the healer. It gives him the courage and strength to handle a violent patient. A mixture from a third bottle is used to wash an unkempt, filthy individual. A client possessed by a devil is sprayed with a different liquid. Another mixture is sprinkled on the eyes and ears of someone suffering from hallucinations. And one more potion is given to the cured patient; appropriately it protects against evil and prevents a relapse.

Magic plays a part in this healer's examination of a patient. He possesses a "magical horn"; it is actually from a goat. For ten to fifteen minutes, it is placed on top of a small mirror. A cord of twisted strings attaches the mirror to a ball approximately six inches in diameter, which is wrapped in a thick twine, and embellished with a few ivory rings. The healer notes that this ball has supernatural powers; in effect, it gives a charge to the horn resting on the mirror.

Once this happens and the horn is infused with magical power, the healer rolls it around the client's head. He moves it across the forehead, above the ears, and allows it to rest on top of the head for a few seconds, presumably to clarify the patient's problem. At this point, the horn is placed in front of the mirror and, according to the healer, a color will be reflected, indicating to him the type of mental illness suffered by the client.

The Kissy healer recognizes four kinds of psychiatric disorder. Each is identified with a color, a model styled from concepts of the ancient world. Black signifies depression; yellow represents a laughing disorder, or schizophrenia; red is mania, and is best typified by a violent person who wants to attack someone; and pink denotes a phobia, an irrational fear, or perhaps a borderline psychosis.

With the diagnosis complete, the treatment process continues. The healer produces four new and different bottles, each containing a special liquid and each related to one of the four categories of madness. The patient drinks a dose from the appropriate bottle. The effect is immediate and quite visible: the client becomes quiet and accessible, and soon takes a nap. Whatever the disorder, this practitioner emphasizes the healing power of rest and sleep. Clearly, his herbal prescriptions facilitate drowsiness, reducing patient anxiety.

He confesses that the most difficult and challenging cases are the depressed and the violent types of mental illness. Claiming success with the sad ones, he notes activity and conversation with people lead to recovery of the depressed. Violent clients frequently require restraint. A wild patient may be placed in chains to prevent escape. The healer informs the client and others that the chains, along with a padlock enveloped in leather, possess special magic and cannot be broken.

In the course of treatment, juju stones, another source of magic, might be used. These are actually two stones, specified as a male and a female, which have been in the healer's family for generations. They have supernatural powers and they pass secret messages to the practitioner. The stones divulge information about the client, indicate the efficacy of the treatment, suggest alternative modes of care, and reveal when a client will be cured. They also may evaluate the moral character of the patient, telling the healer when to terminate the treatment of a bad person.

Near the end of the therapy sessions, several days or weeks after the first interview and when the client appears well on the way to recovery, this healer utilizes a Muslim alpha technique. Taking into consideration the color of a patient's illness, he consults diagrams and a zodiac in an Arabic book in order to find a proper passage from the Koran that will offer consolation to the patient. In the client's presence, he writes in chalk on a slate the Koranic saying, as well as the patient's name. He will then wash the slate clean, collect the liquid, called lasmami, and ask the patient to drink it.

The passage from the Koran may be also written on a piece of paper and folded and placed into a leather container, creating a sebe to be worn around the neck, wrist, or ankle of the client. The final act of the treatment process involves burning the sebe and throwing the ashes into a moving stream. This ritual signifies that a patient has achieved full and complete recovery; now the mental illness has been carried away, and it will never come back.[39]

The Freetown herbalist magician and the Kissy indigenous doctor typify Sierra Leonean traditional practice. Each possesses and demonstrates the qualities of a successful healer: a strong commanding personality, a knowledge of and an ability to exploit herbal medicines, a sensitivity to the dynamics of group conflict, and an awareness and appreciation for the anxiety engendered by fears of unknown, supernatural beings and forces. Each utilizes a basic method of therapy, in which a sort of psychological drama is enacted. The client plays the leading role; the supporting cast includes family and relatives. The healer directs, suggests, reassures, and aims at winning the confidence of the participants.

While herbal remedies are applied, the healer above all seeks to harmonize differences and reintegrate the client into society. An absolute cure to illness is not the overriding aim of therapy. The healer, instead, wants to conserve and restore order within the family and the community. In this way, the group triumphs and overcomes the social and mental troubles of an individual.

This is the thrust of traditional practice. To a large extent, the pattern remains quite uniform throughout the country. Indigenous medicine, however, is very syncretic, and it does adapt and cater to the needs of a particular locale. Where Islamic influences are strong, Muslim alphas take a central part in treating and caring for many of the mentally ill. Some of them specialize in handling psychotic cases. And people believe that alphas are capable of harming as well as helping a distraught person. This power is typically attributed to traditional healers.

While some Temne claim that the alphas use the power of God to cure insanity, they also stress the therapeutics of prayer. Often, a Koranic saying is made into a charm or sebe. Also, verbal inquiries are continued, searching for the social complications of the disorder. And the client may be "smoked out." The client is seated near a container of boiling herbs; a blanket or a cloth is placed over his or her head and the container, allowing the client to inhale the steam, which presumably drives away the evil spirits.

In another area of the country, where secret societies predominate, an important figure in the Poro may be the practitioner. He, too, will have a range of herbal medicines. He may question the patient, diagnose by divination, stage a sacrifice, or receive a confession. He may give a client a counteroath to be applied against some oath of witchcraft. In short, the specifics of traditional practice vary among healers. The essential concerns of therapy, however, remain basic: to mediate conflict and restore balance to the individual and the group.

This social matrix of therapy, combined with the healer's focus on the apparent external agent that has caused the mental illness, accounts largely for the popularity of traditional medicine in Sierra Leone. When a patient becomes violent and intractable or when an indigenous practitioner has failed, the client will be sent to the mental hospital to receive biomedical treatment. Upon discharge from the institution, the patient will return to the care of the traditional healer.

This shunting between hospital and indigenous doctor occurs frequently. Occasionally before being released, a person may be taken out of the hospital by relatives who suspect that a swear or some kind of witchcraft is at the root of a sickness. The client, they feel, requires the attention of a traditional healer, not a psychiatrist.

Such sentiment prevails, and it indicates that for most Sierra Leoneans, biomedicine cannot effectively treat mental disorders. Traditional medicine is preferred and is deemed most suitable for handling the maladies of the mind. This sentiment limits and frustrates the expansion of biomedical psychiatric facilities in the country.

NOTES

1. This information was culled from Kissy Mental Hospital patient record books, 1905-1950.

2. H. U. Ihezue and P. O. Ebigbo, "Present Status and Practice of Electroconvulsive Therapy at the Psychiatric Hospital, Enugu, Nigeria," *Acta Psychiatrica Scandinavica* 63 (1981): 325-32.

3. Selected cases, Kissy Mental Hospital, 1960-1980.

4. Ibid.

5. Interview with director of Kissy Mental Hospital, Dr. E. A. Nahim.

6. Selected cases, Kissy Mental Hospital, 1960-1980.

7. W. G. Jilek, "From Crazy Witch Doctor to Auxiliary Psychotherapist - the Changing Image of the Medicine Man," *Psychiatrica Clinica* 4 (1971): 200-220.

8. Michael Gelfand, *Medicine and Custom in Africa* (Edinburgh: E.and S. Livingstone, 1964); M. J. Field, "Witchcraft as Primitive Interpretation of Mental Disorder," *Journal of Mental Science* 101 (1955); 826-33; Raymond Prince, "Indigenous Yoruba Psychiatry," in Ari Kiev, ed., *Magic, Faith, and Healing: Studies in Primitive Psychiatry Today* (New York: Free Press, 1964), 84-120.

9. C, M. Good, "Traditional Medicine: An Agenda for Medical Geography," *Social Science and Medicine* 11 (1977): 705-13.

10. T. Harding, "Psychosis in a Rural West African Community," *Social Psychiatry* 8 (1973); 198-203.

11. T. Adeoye Lambo, "The Village of Aro," in Maurice King, ed., *Medical Care in Developing Countries* (New York:

Oxford University Press, 1966), 1-7; Lambo, "Experience with a Program in Nigeria," in R. Williams and L. Ozarin, eds., *Community Mental Health: An International Perspective* (San Francisco: Jossey Bass, 1968), 97-110.

12. Herbert Rappaport, "The Tenacity of Folk Psychotherapy: A Functional Interpretation," *Social Psychiatry* 11 (1977): 127-32; Walter Otsyula, "Native and Western Healing: The Dilemma of East African Psychiatry," *Journal of Nervous and Mental Disease* 156 (1973): 297-99; Jeremy R. Dale and David I. Ben-Tovim, "Modern or Traditional? A Study of Treatment Preference for Neuropsychiatric Disorders in Botswana," *British Journal of Psychiatry* 145 (1984): 187-92; M. J. Field, *Search for Security: An Ethno-Psychiatric Study of Rural Ghana* (Evanston, Ill.: Northwestern University Press, 1966); John H. Orley, *Culture and Mental Illness: A Study from Uganda* (Nairobi: East African Publishing House, 1970); I. Sow, *Anthropological Structures of Madness in Black Africa* (New York: International Universities Press, 1980); D. R. Price-Williams, "A Case Study of Ideas Concerning Disease Among the Tiv," *Africa* 32 (1962): 123-31.

13. R. Olukayode Jegede, "A Study of the Role of Socio-Cultural Factors in the Treatment of Mental Illness in Nigeria," *Social Science and Medicine* 15A (1981): 49-54; A. O. Odejide, M. O. Olatawura, Okinade O. Sanda, and A. O. Oyeneye, "Traditional Healers and Mental Illness in the City of Ibadan," *Journal of Black Studies* 9 (1978): 195-205; Gustav Jahoda, "Traditional Healers and Other Institutions Concerned with Mental Illness in Ghana," *International Journal of Social Psychiatry* 7 (1961): 245-68; O. A. Erinosho, "Social Background and Preadmission Sources of Care Among the Yoruba Psychiatric Patients," *Social Psychiatry* 11 (1977): 71-4; Delores E. Mack and G. Tosan-Imade, "The Effects of Ethnicity and Education on Attitudes Toward Mental Illness in Southern Nigeria," *International Journal of Social Psychiatry* 26 (1980): 101-8; Rita Braito and Tolani Asuni, "Traditional Healers in Abeokuta: Recruitment, Professional Affliation, and Types of Patients Healed," in Z. A. Ademuwagun, J.A.A. Ayoade, I. E. Harrison, and D. M. Warren, eds., *African Therapeutic Systems* (Waltham, Mass.: Crossroads Press, 1979), 187-90; Leith Mullings, *Therapy, Ideology, and Social Change: Mental Healing in Urban Ghana* (Berkeley: University of California Press, 1984).

14. Edward C. Green, "Roles for African Traditional Healers in Mental Health Care," *Medical Anthropology* 4 (1980): 489-522; Pascal James Imperato, "Traditional Beliefs and Practices in the City of Timbuctoo," *Bulletin of the New York Acad-*

emy of Medicine 52 (1976): 241-52; Robert B. Edgerton, "A Traditional African Psychiatrist," in David Landy, ed., *Culture, Disease, and Healing: Studies in Medical Anthropology* (New York: Macmillan, 1977), 438-45; Ruth E. Dennis, "The Traditional Healer in Liberia," *Rural Africa* 26 (1974): 17-24; Zacchaeus A. Ademuwagun, "The Relevance of Yoruba Medicine Men in Public Health Practice in Nigeria," *Public Health Reports* 84 (1969): 1085-91; Pascal James Imperato, *African Folk Medicine: Practices and Beliefs of the Bambara and Other Peoples* (Baltimore, Md.: York Press, 1977); Catherine M. Una Maclean, *Magical Medicine* (Edinburgh: University of Edinburgh Press, 1972); Michael Gelfand, "Psychiatric Disorders as Recognized by the Shona," in Ademuwagun, et al., *African Therapeutic Systems*, 176-81.

15. Edward C. Green, "Can Collaborative Programs Between Biomedical and African Indigenous Health Practitioners Succeed?" *Social Science and Medicine* 27 (1988): 1125-30; Amma G. K. Oppong, "Healers in Transition," *Social Science and Medicine* 28 (1989): 605-12; Tolani Asuni, "Modern Medicine and Traditional Medicine," in Ademuwagun, et al., *African Therapeutic Systems*, 176-81.

16. Priscilla R. Ulin, "The Traditional Healer of Botswana in a Changing Society," *Rural Africana* 26 (1974): 123-30; John M. Janzen, *The Quest for Therapy in Lower Zaire* (Berkeley: University of California Press, 1978); P. A. Twumasi, *Medical Systems in Ghana: A Study in Medical Sociology* (Tema, Ghana: Ghana Publishing Corporation, 1975); P. A. Twumasi, "Ashanti Traditional Medicine and Its Relation to Present-Day Psychiatry," in Ademuwagun, et al., *African Therapeutic Systems*, 235-42; Diane Leinwand Zeller, "Traditional and Western Medicine in Buganda: Coexistence and Complement," in Ademuwagun, et al., *African Therapeutic Systems*, 251-58.

17. Ira E. Harrison, "Traditional Healers: A Neglected Source of Manpower," *Rural Africana* 26 (1974): 5-16; David W. Dunlop, "Alternatives to Modern Health Delivery Systems in Africa: Public Policy Issues of Traditional Health Systems," *Social Science and Medicine* 9 (1975): 581-86; Zacchaeus A. Ademuwagun, "Problem and Prospect of Legitimatizing and Integrating Aspects of Traditional Health Care Systems and Methods with Modern Medical Therapy: The Igbo-Ora Experience," in Ademuwagun, et al., *African Therapeutic Systems*, 158-64.

18. Interviews with Dr. E. H. Nahim.

19. Michael Jackson, *The Kuranko: Dimensions of Social Reality in a West African Society* (London: C. Hurst, 1977), 18.

20. Jackson, *The Kuranko*, 39.

21. Robert T. Parsons, *Religion in an African Society: A Study of the Religion of the Kono People of Sierra Leone in Its Social Environment with Special Reference to the Function of Religion in that Society* (Leiden: E. J. Brill, 1963), 19-23.

22. J. G. Edowu Hyde, "The Koranko Perception of Health," *Conference on Health of the Family Unit*, Institute for African Studies, Fourah Bay College, University of Sierra Leone, 17-21 September 1973, 19-23.

23. Jackson, *The Kuranko*, 31-33; Michael D. Jackson, "Structure and Event: Witchcraft Confession Among the Kuranko," *Man* 10 (1975): 387-403.

24. James Steel Thayer, "Native, Culture, and the Supernatural Among the Susu," *American Anthropologist* 10 (1983): 116-32; R. H. Finnegan, *Survey of the Limba People of Northern Sierra Leone* (London: Her Majesty's Stationery Office, 1965): 106-22.

25. Finnegan, *Survey*, 120-22.

26. J.L.M. Dawson,"Traditional Concepts of Mental Health in Sierra Leone," *Sierra Leone Studies*, n.s. 18 (1966-67): 18-19.

27. K. L. Little, *The Mende of Sierra Leone* (London: Routledge and Kegan Paul, 1951); Kenneth Little, "The Mende of Sierra Leone," in *African Worlds: Studies in the Cosmological Ideas and Social Values of African Peoples* (London: Oxford University Press, 1954), 111-37; M. C. Jedrej, "Medicine, Fetish, and Secret Society in West African Culture," *Africa* 46 (1976): 247-57; Dawson, "Traditional Concepts," 19-28.

28. John W. Nunley, *Moving with the Face of the Devil: Art and Politics in Urban West Africa* (Urbana: University of Illinois Press, 1987), 21-23; Leo Spitzer, *The Creoles of Sierra Leone: Responses to Colonialism, 1870-1945* (Madison: University of Wisconsin Press, 1974), 27.

29. Michael Banton, *West African City: A Study of Tribal Life in Freetown* (London: Oxford University Press, 1957), 11-18.

30. Banton, *West African City*, 162-95; Barbara E. Harrell-Bond, Allen M. Howard, and David E. Skinner, *Community Leadership and the Transformation of Freetown, 1801-1976* (The Hague: Mouton Publishers, 1978), 194-95.

31. Harrell-Bond, Howard, and Skinner, *Community Leadership*, 228-32.

32. Banton, *West African City*, 162-95; Kenneth Little, *West African Urbanization: A Study of Voluntary Associations in Social Change* (Cambridge: Cambridge University Press, 1965); John Dawson, "Urbanization and Mental Health in a West African Community," in Kiev, *Magic, Faith, and Healing*, 305-42.

33. Nunley, *Moving with the Face of the Devil*, 38-50.

34. SLA, K 71/40 From Commissioner of Police to the Honourable Colonial Secretary, Juvenile Offenders, 21 February 1941.

35. SLA, CSO K 25/41 Report by Rev. A. Stott on the Nature and Extent of the Problem of Juvenile Delinquency in Sierra Leone.

36. SLA, CSO K 71/30 From the Police Magistrate to the Honourable Colonial Secretary, Juvenile Offenders, 23 January 1940.

37. Nunley, *Moving with the Face of the Devil*, 61-74.

38. Observations and interview with Freetown herbalist magician.

39. Observations and interview with Kissy healer.

7 Conclusion

Sierra Leone, in many ways, represents a microcosm of mental health dilemmas found in most sub-Saharan societies. In common with other African countries, Sierra Leone faces difficult social and environmental problems that frustrate the planning and implementation of health policies and programs. Widespread poverty prevails across the country.

A high mortality rate remains a fundamental feature of Sierra Leonean life. In 1974, life expectancy at birth for females was 45.1 years, and for males, 41.9 years; in the mid-1980s, optimistic estimates set the figures at 50.1 years for women and 46.9 years for men. While the extension of health services may have accounted for a falling death rate, the figures still contrast vividly with the developed world, where life expectancy ranges in the upper seventies for women and the low seventies for men.

The unhealthy status of individuals in Sierra Leone, the waste of human life, is fostered by such debilitating disorders as malaria, helminthiasis, schistosomiasis, and gonococcal infection. According to a 1974 estimate, people under 15 years of age made up 40 percent of the country's population; and they took a disproportionate share of suffering. The chief cause of death among children under 5 years of age include measles, malnutrition, gastroenteritis, neonatal tetanus, bronchopneumonia, and whooping cough. A survey of children in a rural area revealed extremely high instances of anemia, hookworm, and malaria. The report also showed 40 percent of a group of schoolchildren with an enlarged spleen, indicating frequent episodes of malaria. Polio remains most prevalent among children between 5 and 15 years of age, and many of the afflicted end up with a major disability.[1]

Along with poverty and endemic environmental diseases, ig-
norance - notably in regard to corrective hygienic and sanitation
measures - contributes to the poor health conditions. Unaware-
ness about health matters also fosters indifference toward hospitals and dispensaries. A 1982 World Health Organization report
on health in Sierra Leone observed that only 30 percent of the
population used the existing health facilities. Most persons apparently rely on traditional healers, or themselves; they make out by
their own devices, or remain unattended. Many persons accept a
supernatural etiology of both physical and mental disease, a belief
that further insulates them from the offerings of modern medicine. Public health in Sierra Leone has also been affected by low
government expenditures on medical services, a situation exacerbated by a weak and inflationary economy.[2]

The end result of these circumstances for mental health programs remains a foregone conclusion evident throughout this
analysis: in a poor environment ravaged by infectious diseases,
mental health issues seem insignificant and of minor practical importance. Limited government resources and funds are directed
toward resolving urgent and immediate matters such as providing
comfort and relief from malaria, nutritional deficiency diseases,
and parasite infections.

While the government has hesitated to invest significantly in
psychiatric care and treatment, or to embark on new mental
health programs, this does not mean that the presumption found
in the writings of Western observers is true. Medical analyses of
Third World psychiatric services frequently assert that effective
care and treatment is provided to a small minority of patients and
that the majority of mentally distressed persons remained un-
treated. These individuals, it is claimed, are detected and incarcerated only after posing a threat to community order and
safety.[3]

This assumption that a few benefit and the majority suffer
overlooks the work of traditional medical practitioners. In Sierra
Leone, and across Africa, largely in urban areas, differing
therapeutic systems - traditional healers with various treatment
options, along with the practitioners of Western medicine - compete, coexist, and interact. A pluralistic view prevails regarding
the management, control, and cure of the mentally disordered.
The involvement of the government in programs for the mentally
ill, its funding of a mental hospital, for example, represents only
one indicator of psychiatric care, since traditional healers play a
major role in the country's mental health system.

Yet over the years, the mental hospital in Sierra Leone has remained a significant institution that reflects the social problems of the wider society. Its origins had a significance related to the founding of the colony. A humanitarian, utopian goal figured prominently in the establishment of the early Freetown settlements: the area served as a place for refuge for ex-slaves from Africa and England as well as the New World.

In like manner, altruism influenced the creation of the insane asylum at Kissy. A unique situation demanded resolution. Former slaves displaying erratic and socially disruptive behavior could not be allowed to run about Freetown. Many were recent arrivals; they were without family or friends and quite removed from their original home, village, or country. For these reasons, an institution of refuge, an insane asylum, became a necessity. While serving as a haven for poor, insane ex-slaves, it functioned as an agency for controlling a potentially difficult social problem.

In another way, the Kissy mental institution had a unique beginning. Unlike many African facilities for the mentally ill, it emerged from a hospital, not a prison, and it remained, throughout its history, under the supervision of medical authorities. In contrast to Kissy, for example, Zomba Lunatic Asylum in colonial Nyasaland, the area of present-day Malawi, was established in 1910 as a wing of the central prison, and until 1951, it was a custodial correctional facility under the direction of the colony's department of prisons. In 1955, Zomba's first psychiatrist was appointed to administer the institution.[4]

Many other sub-Saharan facilities for the insane had origins similar to the Malawi institution. In mid-nineteenth century British Nigeria, a ward for the mentally ill was maintained at Lagos prison. The demands of prison authorities for the removal of non-criminal lunatics, coupled with the increasingly overcrowded conditions, encouraged the development of plans for other institutions for the mentally disordered and led to the opening of Yaba Lunatic Asylum in 1907.[5]

Welfare and correctional concerns were most evident in the beginnings of mental health care in South Africa. At Capetown, the British provided hospitals for sick paupers. Old Somerset Hospital accepted all kinds of incapacitated persons, including lunatics. And facilities on Robben Island, a remote convict settlement, served as a depository for insane persons sent from various jails. Late in the nineteenth century, when mental institutions appeared throughout the country, the Robben Island unit became a hospital.[6]

Similar patterns of development were evident in other parts of the British Empire, notably at two widely different island settlements, Barbados and Tasmania. Until 1893, when Barbados Mental Hospital was constructed, the mentally ill on this Caribbean island were kept in varied settings, including almshouses, jails, and a building designated as a lunatic asylum.[7] In Tasmania, a facility housing pauper invalids and lunatics became a mental hospital in 1848. Over the years, it offered care to three kinds of patients: the criminally insane, the mentally retarded, and the mentally ill.[8]

Throughout the nineteenth century, British India had a special arrangement for the mentally ill in a segregated system, a dual set of institutions that physically separated the Indian, or native, from the European, largely English, clientele. The control of social disorder, of persons displaying erratic and violent behavior, was a prominent concern behind the creation of the dual hospital system. Authorities were alarmed about criminals and mischievous persons wandering about the community disturbing peace and order. By 1850, a number of native lunatic asylums had been established in the provincial towns; and asylums for the European insane were maintained in the large cities of Calcutta, Bombay, and Madras.

The institutionalization of the European mad had a certain significance. The British community in India was divided along very distinct class lines. The elite adopted an exclusive and aristocratic life-style, and looked down on the poorer classes, who made up the majority of Europeans in the colony. These poorer persons often displayed manners that seemed obnoxious, reckless, or licentious to the elite: and such behavior, the authorities argued, damaged the image of the Europeans. Psychiatric confinement of a disruptive and undesirable mentally ill English person conveniently removed an embarrassment to the ruling power. It facilitated the acceptance and the maintenance of colonial authority and order.[9]

From this brief overview of the origins of mental institutions throughout the British Empire in the nineteenth century, a basic pattern emerges. This model relates closely to the historical experience of institutionalizing insane people in Europe, as described by Michel Foucault, Klaus Doerner, Andrew Scull, and Vieda Skultans.[10] The social control of an unreliable or unpredictable element of the population provided a rationale, an initial purpose, for establishing a psychiatric institution. This concern was often couched in humanitarian or medical terminology, and a certain practical altruism was evident. Yet the overriding perception and intention remained: persons acting in socially disruptive ways were deemed a threat to the community and required incarceration in a special facility. Local circumstances determined the kind of institution. It could be a jail, an almshouse, or a hospital, or a facility of mixed character that combined the features of correctional as well as a welfare agency.

As the Kissy asylum in Sierra Leone illustrates, local conditions also regulated an institution's target population. For example, initially the majority of clients at Kissy were recently arrived ex-slaves living in Freetown and the surrounding area; for a long time, only a few patients were sent from other parts of the country. While these inmates remained unique to Sierra Leone, and every other mental institution on the continent had its own specific and local types of patients, mental hospitals throughout Africa served a common, general clientele - namely, socially marginal and economically deprived persons, who over time greatly increased in numbers and were largely outside the occupational system. Many were unemployed, unskilled, and frequently transient people; varied kinds of criminals formed an additional segment of this patient population. They came from the large and growing amorphous class of the urban poor, who madeup a major part of the culture of the tropical towns and cities of Africa.

In the twentieth century, notably since World War II, rural-urban migration became a massive movement. Cities drew people from the hinterlands searching for jobs, goods, schools, and amenities - in short, the stimulation, opportunities, and challenges of urban life. A few achieved success - many did not - and the migration persisted. City populations doubled in less than fifteen years; Ibadan, Nigeria trebled in twenty years. Large concentrations of people gathered in shantytowns and slums in the fringes of such cities as Nairobi, Abidjan, Accra, Lagos, and Freetown.

In these settings, people lived under conditions that nourished pathology. They stayed in overcrowded, unsanitary hovels without adequate water or sewage facilities. Tattered sheets or blankets covered doorways and window frames; children crawled in uncollected rubbish and sewage drains; the hot climate fostered the growth of flies, snails, and mosquitos. Here perhaps more than in the country, malaria, tuberculosis, bilharziasis, helminthiasis, and other infectious diseases abounded; malnutrition and accompanying deficiency disorders were common.[11]

In addition to living under such physical conditions, the urban poor were caught in a stressful psychosocial milieu. Unemployment remained the basic fact of life. The few available jobs were always overwhelmed with too many applicants; police discouraged any effort to subsist by hawking. The poverty-stricken migrant sought support and aid from familial, ethnic, and voluntary associations. This help eased some of the stresses confronting the urban poor, but over time, the affiliations eroded under the pressure of deprivation and poverty.

Without any continual network of support, the unemployed stood alone, removed from the familiar and traditional patterns of life. Adrift from home, village, family, relatives, and friends, social isolation and alienation grew. The migrant became part of a disorganized social matrix, a disruptive and complex social order of diverse ethnic and linguistic groups. This was a threatening and insecure environment disposed toward physical and psychosocial pathology. Many of the migrants, particularly the unprotected and those ill-equipped to cope with the ways of the city, pursued illicit activities. They succumbed to alcoholism or drug abuse, or entered prostitution, or engaged in varied forms of social disorder. Some became mentally ill.[12]

A major disruptive feature of this social setting was an excess of young males, either single or married but without their families. Since colonial times, their ranks had swollen increasingly, and authorities remained apprehensive about the potential for disorder and violence perpetrated by unemployed young men. A few were prone to violence: they formed gangs and fought the police and each other for territory, and often preyed on squatter areas. While poverty was the root cause of this antisocial behavior and delinquency, most of the urban poor, female as well as male, were nonviolent. Crime, across the continent, as in Sierra Leone, was chiefly against property. Petty theft was most common; it was the way some people eked out an existence. Stealing, along with begging and hawking, were the means of survival in the harsh world of the urban poor.[13]

When the majority of clients to Kissy Mental Hospital and other African mental institutions began to come out of this urban underclass, the link between mental and social disorders became most apparent. As noted earlier, this has been a recent development. Throughout the nineteenth century, traditional authorities and healers coped with the mentally ill and socially disruptive members of their communities. They were restrained, observed, and treated within family structures or special compounds designed for reintegrating sick people into community life.

As time went by, notably after World War II, urban centers underwent rapid growth; a greater variety of social problems developed, and were manifested most dramatically on the streets and in the poorer housing districts of the large cities. Here, the increased incidence of marital troubles, alcoholism, drug dependence, and crime have led to more displays of antisocial, and at times violent and psychotic behavior. Authorities often send to mental hospitals individuals exhibiting erratic and disruptive conduct. In many cases, such behavior is symptomatic of a social rather than a mental disorder.

In addition, the irreducible quota of vagrant psychotics, an element of the urban poor, has increased in number and has precipitated a social problem common to African cities and towns. These persons wander about naked or unsuitably dressed. They talk to themselves, chase animals, sleep in streets, throw stones at people and buildings, and collect rubbish. They might have abused others, sung and danced in market places, or stolen food and articles from vendors. A few are elderly and mentally retarded, or have physical infirmities. The majority were diagnosed as schizophrenic, undifferentiated type, when they were incarcerated in a mental institution.

Vagrant psychotics are distinguished from beggars and the destitute chiefly by their conduct. During their time of arrest and detention, they display aberrant behavior, which leads to their referral for psychiatric observation and assessment. In recent years, authorities have viewed vagrants as embarrassments to the society and have forcibly removed them from the streets, notably when important persons or large numbers of tourists are evident.[14]

While destitute and sometimes unruly persons madeup a portion of the clients of African mental hospitals, still other features characterized patient populations.[15] In contrast to Western institutions, males outnumbered females. At some facilities, a three-to-one ratio prevailed; at most places, there were two men to every woman. This preponderance of male mental patients may be attributed largely to the acceptance of traditional sex roles. As the breadwinner, the African man cannot afford to be sick for an extended time period; his earnings remain vital to the support and survival of the family. A mentally disturbed man receives hospital treatment, then, to curtail loss of income.

Unemployed single men, however, form a major part of the patient population. Their tendency to act out inner conflict, to resort to aggressive or violent behavior, constitutes a threat to social order and requires incarceration in an institution. Women, on the other hand, have generally remained in the home, where mental illness can be tolerated and controlled. Relatives want a woman's madness kept private, realizing that public awareness of familial insanity diminishes her chances for marriage.

Along with males prevailing over females, another common feature in African mental facilities has been the predominance of young persons, economically deprived and largely unschooled. This contrasts with Western institutions, which hold a much older patient population. In line with a pattern in America and Europe, however, there was a noticeable age and marital difference distinguishing the sexes. In most psychiatric categories, as well as among the nondesignated cases, the majority of patients included single men and married older women. Some of the men and women were divorced or separated from spouse or family. Again, Sierra Leone was typical.

There were other distinctions between the sexes. Neurotic disorder seemed more prevalent among women than men. And a gendered symptomatology has been revealed. Women complained about aches and pains, about feeling sad, and, at times, tense. In contrast, men tended to be agitated, aggressive, or disoriented, and often hypochondriacal. On the other hand, gender was not a primary factor determining the utilization of psychiatric services. Better-educated and more affluent people turned to psychiatry when faced with a problem of mental disorder. The poorer and less-trained individual went to the traditional healer.

The nature of mental illness in Sierra Leone, and throughout sub-Saharan Africa, remains comparable to that in the developed areas of the world. Schizophrenia represented the most prominent disorder. At some facilities, it accounted for 70 percent of admissions. Organic psychoses were common and often associated with infections and drug intoxications, as well as meningitis and encephalitis. Mental deficiency, epilepsy, puerperal psychosis, and personality disorders were represented in small samples. Affective disorders were prominent, affirming the more recent reports and studies showing widespread depression among Africans. In short, the various types of mental disorder recognized in the West have been recorded in Africa. African psychiatrists confidently assert that the psychoses found in the Western world are evident, and, in some instances, more prevalent in the Third World.

A high incidence of acute transient psychosis remains a psychiatric disorder unique to Africa and the developing world. Many observers insist that this is a psychiatric disorder peculiar to a society in a state of flux - a society where traditional and conservative values and roles have faded and no longer seem important, or are in conflict with a new order that has an uncertain and indeterminate future. Other researchers attribute acute psychotic episodes to physiological disturbances brought on by infections, parasitism, vitamin deficiency, malnutrition, and other states rampant in a culture of poverty and insufficient health care. And cultural attitudes are important: African societies have a wide tolerance for displays of emotional reactions to pain and distress.

In addition to short-lived transient psychotic reactions, many medical observers view the somatic symptoms of African mental patients as a psychiatric expression unique to underdeveloped areas. Somatic complaints in depression, they assert, demonstrate that the affective psychoses are widespread in Africa. What remains important here, however, is not the number or the quality of culture-bound syndromes, but the relevance of psychiatry to the developing world.

Today, African psychiatrists are eclectic and have an exceedingly practical turn of mind. They believe psychiatry can account for the majority of African mental disorders; in itself, however, psychiatry cannot resolve or control or diminish the mental health problems of the Third World. While it represents an important way, or perhaps a tool or method, of detecting mental illness and coping with mental distress, local values as well as socioeconomic and demographic conditions play the decisive role in African mental health care. Not least is the factor so constant in Sierra Leone: governments deal with tight budgets and depleted funds and officials remain unconvinced of the importance of investing in psychiatric services and facilities.

Aside from this difficult political issue, a basic personnel problem persists: the diminishing proportion of persons providing health care. And distressing and painful social problems, namely, poverty, famine, unemployment, drug abuse, and family breakdown, erode the lives of individuals and communities. These fundamental social dilemmas must be addressed and eased before any major improvement in mental health care can be effected.

Over the years, Kissy Mental Hospital has endured and prevailed; it has displayed remarkable resilience. The societal and political limitations imposed on the institution have been offset by its essential, humane, and adaptive role in meeting the needs of its clientele. To be sure, throughout its history, the custodial function has remained paramount. Often this policy has dealt solely with maintaining the physical condition of the patients: this has meant treating a sickness such as malaria or tuberculosis, or combatting malnutrition, or caring for an accident injury rather than alleviating some psychiatric impairment. In addition to attending to the physical health of patients, hospital administrators have adopted programs that reflected the therapeutics of Western psychiatric features. For example, the psychopharmaceutical treatments utilized in the mental hospitals of the United Kingdom have also been used at the Kissy institution.

In recent years, the hospital leadership has promoted community mental health programs aimed at preventing the long-term institutionalization of mental patients. Under this policy, clients are admitted for a limited time period; the family is required to remain in contact with their incarcerated relative; and criminal cases are no longer imposed on or accepted by the hospital. These initiatives are complemented with a community outreach policy that encourages and supports the mental health work of religious groups and organizations, as well as of traditional healers. In short, today, Kissy Mental Hospital, beset with problems and dilemmas as throughout its history, remains a vital part of the medical system of Sierra Leone. The dedication, flexibility, and compassion of its current leadership exemplifies the best of African psychiatry.

NOTES

1. Carol P. MacCormack, "Primary Health Care in Sierra Leone," *Social Science and Medicine* 19 (1984): 199-208; A. Raymond Mills, "The Effects of Urbanization on Health in a Mining Area of Sierra Leone," *Transactions of the Royal Society of Tropical Medicine and Hygiene* 61 (1967): 114-30; Borbor Sama Kandeh, "Causes of Infant and Early Childhood Death in Sierra Leone," *Social Science and Medicine* 23 (1986): 297-303; David P. Gamble, "Infant Mortality Rates in a Sierra Leonean Urban Community (Lunsar)," *Journal of Tropical Medicine and Hygiene* 64 (1961): 192-99; Franklyn Lisk and Rolph Van Der Hoeven, "Measurement and Interpretation of Poverty in Sierra Leone," *International Labor Review* 118 (1979): 713-30; Carolyn Adcock, "Poliomyelitis in Sierra Leone," *British Medical Journal* 285 (1982): 1031-32.

2. *Sierra Leone Country Profile (Health)* (Geneva: World Health Organization, 2nd edition, 1982).

3. Timothy W. Harding, "Psychiatry in Rural Agrarian Societies," *Psychiatric Annals* 8 (1978): 302-10.

4. Megan Vaughan, "Idioms of Madness: Zomba Lunatic Asylum, Nyasaland, in the Colonial Period," *Journal of Southern*

African Studies 9 (1983): 218-38.

5. Alexander Boroffka, "Mental Illness in Lagos: History of the Yaba Mental Hospital from 1907 to 1966," *Psychopathologie Africaine* 9 (1973): 405-17.

6. John Iliffe, *The African Poor: A History* (London: Cambridge University Press, 1987), 102-7; Lewis A. Hurst and Mary B. Lucas, "South Africa," in John G. Howells, ed., *World History of Psychiatry* (New York: Brunner/Mazel, 1975), 600-623.

7. Lawrence E. Fisher, *Colonial Madness: Mental Health in the Barbadian Social Order* (New Brunswick, N.J.: Rutgers University Press, 1985).

8. John C. Burnham, "The Royal Derwent Hospital in Tasmania: Historical Perspectives on the Meaning of Community Psychiatry," *Australian and New Zealand Journal of Psychiatry* 9 (1975): 163-68.

9. Waltraud Ernst, "The Establishment of Native Lunatic Asylums in Early Nineteenth Century British India," in G. Jan Meulenbeld and Dominik Wujastyk, eds., *Studies on Indian Medical History* (Groningen, The Netherlands: Egbert Forsten, 1987), 169-204; Waltraud Ernst, "The European Insane in British India, 1800-1858: A Case Study of Psychiatry and Colonial Rule," in David Arnold, ed., *Imperial Medicine and Indigenous Societies* (Manchester: Manchester University Press, 1989), 27-44.

10. Michel Foucault, *Madness and Civilization* (New York: Vintage Books, 1973); Klaus Doerner, *Madmen and the Bourgeoisie* (Oxford: Basil Blackwell, 1981); Andrew T. Scull, *Museums of Madness* (New York: St. Martin's Press, 1979); Vieda Skultans, *English Madness: Ideas on Insanity 1580-1890* (London: Routledge and Kegan Paul, 1979).

11. Iliffe, *The African Poor*, 164-92, 230-59; Charles C. Hughes and John M. Hunter, "Disease and Development in Africa," *Social Science and Medicine* 3 (1970): 443-68.

12. Hughes and Hunter, "Disease and Development in Africa," 468-93; Peter C. W. Gutkind, "The Energy of Despair: Social Organization of the Unemployed in Two African Cities: Lagos and Nairobi," *Civilization* 17 (1967): 186-214, 380-405.

13. Iliffe, *The African Poor*, 137-38, 165, 175-76, 188-89, 244-45.

14. T. Asuni, *Vagrant Psychotics in Abeokuta* (Abeokuta, Nigeria, unpublished paper, 1971); A. O. Odejide, "Chronic Psychotic Patients in Nigeria: Adverse Prognostic Factors," *International Journal of Social Psychiatry* 28 (1982): 213-22.

15. This social and psychiatric characterization of African mental patients is culled from a variety of sources, notably: Adebayo Olabisi Odejide, Lamidi Kolawole Oyewunmi, and Jude

Uzoma Ohaeri, "Psychiatry in Africa: An Overview," *American Journal of Psychiatry* 146 (1989): 708-16; G. Allen German, "Mental Health in Africa: II. The Nature of Mental Disorder in Africa Today. Some Clinical Observations," *British Journal of Psychiatry* 151 (1987): 440-46; Wilbert M. Giesler and E. A. Nahim, "Client Characteristics at Kissy Mental Hospital, Freetown, Sierra Leone," *Social Science and Medicine* 18 (1984): 819-25; "Mental Health in Developing Countries," *British Medical Journal* 4 (1975): 187-88; Tsung-Yi Lin, "Mental Health in the Third World," *Journal of Nervous and Mental Disease* 171 (1983): 71-78; R. Giel and T. Harding, "Psychiatric Problems in Developing Countries," *British Journal of Psychiatry* 123 (1976): 513-22; T. W. Harding, M. V. De Arongo, J. Baltazar, C. E. Climent, H.H.A. Ibrahim, C. Ladrido-Ignacio, R. Shrinivasa Murthy, and N. N. Wig, "Mental Disorders in Primary Health Care: A Study of Their Frequency and Diagnosis in Four Developing Countries," *Psychological Medicine* 10 (1980): 231-41; David I. Ben-Tovim, "DSI-III in Botswana: A Field Trial in a Developing Country," *American Journal of Psychiatry* 142 (1985): 342-45; U. H. Ihezue, "Some Observations and Comments on the Psychosocial Profile of First-ever Referrals to the Psychiatric Hospital, Enugu, Nigeria," *Acta Psychiatrica Scandinavica* 65 (1982): 355-64; G.G.C. Rwegellera and C. C. Mambwe, "Diagnostic Classification of First-ever Admissions to Chainama Hills Hospital, Lusaka, Zambia," *British Journal of Psychiatry* 130 (1977): 573-80; Charles R. Swift and Tolani Asuni, *Mental Health and Disease in Africa: With Special Reference to Africa South of the Sahara* (Edinburgh: Churchill Livingstone, 1975); G. M. Carstairs, "Psychiatric Problems in Developing Countries," *British Journal of Psychiatry* 123 (1973): 271-77; U. H. Ihezue and N. Kumaraswamy, "A Psychosocial Study of Igbo Schizophrenic Patients Treated at a Nigerian Psychiatric Hospital," *Acta Psychiatrica Scandinavica* 70 (1984): 310-15; U. H. Ihezue, "Psychiatric In-Patients in Anambra State, Nigeria," *Acta Psychiatrica Scandinavica* 68 (1983): 277-86; Joop T.V.M. DeJong, Guus A. J. DeKlein, and Sineke G.H.H.M. Ten Horn, "A Baseline Study of Mental Disorders in Guine-Bissau," *British Journal of Psychiatry* 148 (1986): 27-32; R. Olukayode Jegede, "Outpatient Psychiatry in an Urban Clinic in a Developing Country," *Social Psychiatry* 13 (1978): 93-9; A. Binitie, "Outcome of Neurotic Disorders in African Patients," *Acta Psychiatrica Scandinavica* 63 (1981): 110-16; A. Binite, "Psychiatric Disorders in a Rural Practice in the Bendel State of Nigeria," *Acta Psychiatrica Scandinavica* 64 (1981): 273-80; L. Jacobsson, "Mental Disorders Admitted to a General Hospital in Western Ethiopia, 1960-1970," *Acta Psychiatrica Scandinavica*

71 (1985): 410-16; L. Jacobsson, "Psychiatric Morbidity and Psychosocial Background in an Outpatient Population of a General Hospital in Western Ethiopia," *Acta Psychiatrica Scandinavica* 71 (1985): 417-26; W.P.J.C. Onyeama, "Social and Clinical Features of Patients at a State Psychiatric Hospital in Nigeria," in Olayiwola A. Erinosho and Norman W. Bell, eds., *Mental Health in Africa* (Ibadan: Ibadan University Press, 1982), 122-29; David M. Ndetei and Joseph Muhangi, "The Prevalence and Clinical Presentation of Psychiatric Illness in a Rural Setting in Kenya," *British Journal of Psychiatry* 135 (1979): 269-72; David I. Ben-Tovim and Josephine M. Cushnie, "The Prevalence of Schizophrenia in a Remote Area of Botswana," *British Journal of Psychiatry* 148 (1986): 576-80; J. C. Vyncke, "The Psychiatric Service of the General Hospital Prince Regent Charles at Usumbura (Ruanda-Urundi), Africa," in *Frontiers of General Hospital Psychiatry* (New York: International University Press, 1961), 430-37; E. D. Wittkower and L. Bijou, "Psychiatry in Developing Countries," *American Journal of Psychiatry* 120 (1963): 218-21.

Bibliographical Essay

What follows is a commentary on the most important sources utilized for this book. It is a selective bibliography and not an exhaustive compilation of all materials on the subject.

Much of this study rests on unpublished primary sources located in Sierra Leone, that is, in the Kissy Mental Hospital and in the National Archives of Sierra Leone. A major part of these materials includes the records of mental patients at the Kissy institution. Over four thousand individual case histories were examined; and while some gaps in this data exist - for example, religious affiliation, occupation, and ethnic identity were not always specified - the bulk of the information in these records remains a resource rich with vital statistics and demographic details, as well as medical observations on aberrant mental and social behavior.

The sources used from the National Archives of Sierra Leone embrace a wide range of items, including the annual reports of the medical department of the colonial government (some are handwritten documents), as well as memos, directives, reports, commentaries, and letters of colonial officials. Other papers are from relatives of mental patients and from community and religious leaders concerned with the care and treatment of the mentally ill.

Most of the archival materials deal with the practical problems of operating a mental hospital - maintaining the physical plant, controlling admissions and discharges, establishing treatment regimens, coping with violent clients, preventing the escapes of inmates, and disciplining staff for maltreating patients.

An impressive and growing bibliography on the history of Sierra Leone is readily available. Some of the more important studies include: Christopher Fyfe, *A History of Sierra Leone* (London: Oxford University Press, 1962); C. Magbaily Fyle, *The History of Sierra Leone* (London: Evans Brothers, 1981); Leo Spitzer, *The Creoles of Sierra Leone: Responses to Colonialism, 1870-1945* (Madison: University of Wisconsin Press, 1974); Akintola J. G. Wyse, "Some Thoughts on Sierra Leone History," *Journal of the Historical Society of Sierra Leone* 2 (Jan. 1978): 1-9; Akintola Wyse, *The Krio of Sierra Leone: An Interpretive History* (Freetown: Okrafo-Smart, 1989); Cyril P. Foray, *Historical Dictionary of Sierra Leone* (Metuchen, N.J.: Scarecrow Press, 1977); Martin Kilson, *Political Change in a West African State: A Study of the Modernization Process in Sierra Leone* (New York: Atheneum, 1969); Murray Last, Paul Richards, and Christopher Fyfe, eds., *Sierra Leone 1787-1987: Two Centuries of Intellectual Life* (Manchester: Manchester University Press, 1987; Joe A. D. Alie, *A New History of Sierra Leone* (New York: St. Martin's Press, 1990).

On the growth of Freetown see, Barbara E. Harrell-Bond, Allen M. Howard, and David E. Skinner, *Community Leadership and the Transformation of Freetown, 1801-1976* (The Hague: Mouton Publishers, 1978); Michael Banton, *West African City: A Study of Tribal Life in Freetown* (London: Oxford University Press, 1957); Christopher Fyfe and Eldred Jones, *Freetown: A Symposium* (Freetown: Sierra Leone University Press, 1968).

Only a few historical works exist on the far-reaching subjects of mental health care and mental illness in sub-Saharan Africa. A good article is Megan Vaughan, "Idioms of Madness: Zomba Lunatic Asylum, Nyasaland, in the Colonial Period," *Journal of Southern African Studies* 9 (1983): 218-38. Other works, written by clinicians and having a limited historical perspective, are *Mental Disorders and Mental Health in Africa South of the Sahara* (Geneva: World Health Organization, 1958); Alexander Boroffka, "Mental Illness in Lagos: History of the Yaba Mental Hospital from 1907 to 1966," *Psychopathologie Africaine* 9 (1973): 405-17; John G. Howells, ed., *World History of Psychiatry* (New York: Brunner/Mazel, 1975); Olayiwola A. Erinosho, "The Evolution of Modern Psychiatric Care in Nigeria," *American Journal of Psychiatry* 136 (1979): 1572-75; Olayiwola A. Erinosho and Norman W. Bell, eds., *Mental Health in Africa* (Ibadan: Ibadan University Press, 1982); D. M. Ndetei, "Psychiatry in Kenya: Yesterday, Today, and Tomorrow," *Acta Psychiatrica Scandinavica* 62 (1980): 210-11.

A major historical study on German psychiatry in Africa is Albert Diefenbacher, *Psychiatrie und Kolonialismus: Zur "Irrenfürsorge in der Kolonie Deutsch-Ostafrika* (Frankfurt: Campus Verlag, 1985). For a French perspective, see Henri Collomb, "Histoire de la psychiatrie en Afrique noire francophone," *African Journal of Psychiatry* 2 (1975): 87-115; Antonine Porot, "L'oeuvre psychiatrique de la France aux colonies depuis un siècle," *Annales Médico-Psychologiques* 101 (1943): 357-78.

In contrast to the paucity of historical analyses, a large number of studies on African mental illness and mental health care can be found in the medical and psychiatric literature. A selective list includes: Adebayo Olabisi Odejide, Lamidi Kolawole Oyewunmi, and Jude Uzoma Ohaeri, "Psychiatry in Africa: An Overview," *American Journal of Psychiatry* 146 (1989): 708-16; G. Allen German, "Mental Health in Africa: I. The Extent of Mental Health Problems in Africa Today. An Update of Epidemiological Knowledge," *British Journal of Psychiatry* 151 (1987): 435-39; German, "Mental Health in Africa: II. The Nature of Mental Disorder in Africa Today. Some Clinical Observations," *British Journal of Psychiatry* 151 (1987): 440-46; German, "Aspects of Clinical Psychiatry in sub-Saharan Africa," *British Journal of Psychiatry* 121 (1972): 461-79; G. M. Carstairs, "Psychiatric Problems in Developing Countries," *British Journal of Psychiatry* 123 (1973): 271-77. An excellent text is Charles R. Swift and Tolani Asuni, *Mental Health and Disease in Africa: With Special Reference to Africa South of the Sahara* (Edinburgh: Churchill Livingstone, 1975). Each of the above sources provides a substantial bibliography.

The best guides to medical sources in the periodical literature are the *Index Catalogue of the Library of the Surgeon-General's Office* and the *Index Medicus*. African medical journals offer very relevant and useful information, notably *East African Medical Journal, Central African Journal of Medicine, African Journal of Medical Science, African Journal of Psychiatry, Ghana Medical Journal, Nigerian Medical Journal*, and *West African Medical Journal*. Two other professional journals, *Journal of Tropical Medicine* and *Psychopathologie Africaine*, as well as the reports and proceedings of the Pan-African Psychiatric Conferences, are essential sources.

The writings of the Nigerian psychiatrist T. Adeoye Lambo remain central to any discussion on recent African psychiatry. Some examples of Lambo's research include: "The Role of Cultural Factors in Paranoid Psychoses among the Yoruba Tribe,"

Journal of Mental Science 101 (1955): 239-66; "Neuropsychiatric Observations in the Western Regions of Nigeria," *British Medical Journal* 2 (1956): 1388-94; "Further Neuropsychiatric Observations in Nigeria," *British Medical Journal* 11 (1960): 1696-1704; "Malignant Anxiety: A Syndrome Associated with Criminal Conduct in Africans," *Journal of Mental Science* 108 (1962): 256-64; "Adolescents Transplanted from Their Traditional Environment: Problems and Lessons out of Africa,"*Clinical Pediatrics* 6 (1967): 438-45; "Neuro-psychiatric Syndromes Associated with Human Trypanosomiasis in Tropical Africa," *Acta Psychiatrica Scandinavica* 42 (1966): 474-84; "The Village of Aro," in Maurice King, ed., *Medical Care in Developing Countries* (New York: Oxford University Press, 1966), 1-7; "Experience with a Program in Nigeria," in R. Williams and L. Ozarin, eds., *Community Mental Health: An International Perspective* (San Francisco: Jossey Bass, 1968).

Lambo was also one of the authors of a classic ethno- or cross-cultural psychiatric study: A. M. Leighton, T. A. Lambo, C. C. Hughes, D. C. Leighton, J. M. Murphy, and D. B. Macklin, *Psychiatric Disorder Among the Yoruba* (Ithaca, N.Y.: Cornell University Press, 1963. Other related transcultural works are M. J. Field, *Search for Security: An Ethno-Psychiatric Study of Rural Ghana* (Evanston, Ill.: Northwestern University Press, 1966); John H. Orley, *Culture and Mental Illness: A Study from Uganda* (Nairobi: East African Publishing House, 1970); and I. Sow, *Anthropological Structures of Madness in Black Africa* (New York: International Universities Press, 1980).

Over the years, the perceptions of madness in Africa have changed. A good article illustrating the evolving views on depression is Raymond Prince, "The Changing Picture of Depressive Syndromes in Africa," *Canadian Journal of African Studies* 1 (1968): 177-92. A sample of recent research includes: M. Diop, "La dépression chez le noir africain," *Psychopathologie Africaine* 3 (1967): 183-94; T. Buchan, "Depression in African Patients," *South African Medical Journal* 43 (1969): 1055-58; D. M. Ndetei and A. Vadher, "Types of Life Events Associated with Depression in a Kenyan Setting," *Acta Psychiatrica Scandinavica* 66 (1982): 163-68; O. I. Ifabumuyi, "Demographic Characteristics of Depressives in Northern Nigeria," *Acta Psychiatrica Scandinavica* 68 (1983): 271-76; U. H. Ihezue and N. Kumaraswamy, "Socio-Demographic Factors of Depressive Illness Among Nigerians," *Acta Psychiatrica Scandinavica* 73 (1986): 128-32. Two excellent cross-cultural perspectives on depression are: Arthur Kleinman and Byron Good, eds., *Culture and Depression* (Berkeley: University of California Press, 1985), and Arthur Kleinman, *Social Origins of Distress and Disease: Depression, Neurasthenia, and Pain in Modern China* (New Haven: Yale University Press, 1986).

Good examples of British medical opinion on African mental illness in the colonial era are T. Duncan Greenlees, "Insanity among the Natives of South Africa," *Journal of Mental Science* 41 (1895): 71-79; R. Howard, "Emotional Psychoses Among Dark-Skinned Races," *Journal of Tropical Medicine and Hygiene* 13 (1910): 169-73; N. Dembovitz, "Psychiatry Among West African Troops," *Journal of the Royal Army Medical Corps* 84 (1945): 70-74; J. C. Carothers, *The African Mind in Health and Disease: A Study in Ethnopsychiatry* (Geneva: World Health Organization, 1953). Two detailed reports came out of the late colonial period: R. Cunyngham Brown, *Report III: On the Care and Treatment of Lunatics in the British West African Colonies: Nigeria* (Lagos 1938); and Geoffrey Tooth, *Studies in Mental Illness in the Gold Coast* (London: His Majesty's Stationery Office, 1950).

In recent years, many studies have dealt with the sociology of African mental illness. This literature develops several themes. On cultural conflict, see Ronald M. Wintrob, "A Study of Disillusionment: Depressive Reactions of Liberian Students Returning from Advance Training Abroad," *American Journal of Psychiatry* 123 (1967): 1593-97; M. Assael and G. A. German, "Changing Society and Mental Health in Eastern Africa," *Israel Annals of Psychiatry and Related Disciplines* 8 (1970): 52-74; Morton Beiser and Henri Collomb, "Mastering Change: Epidemiological and Case Studies in Senegal, West Africa," *American Journal of Psychiatry* 138 (1981): 455-59; Henri Collomb and Henry Ayats, "Les migration au Sénégal: étude psychopathologique," *Cahiers d'Etudes Africaines* 2 (1962): 570-97. There are several good sociological reports focusing on rural settings: R. Giel and J. N. Van Luijk, "Psychiatric Morbidity in a Small Ethiopian Town," *British Journal of Psychiatry* 115 (1969): 149-62; John Orley and John K. Wing, "Psychiatric Disorders in Two African Villages," *Archives of General Psychiatry* 36 (1979): 513-20; M. J. Field, "Mental Disorder in Rural Ghana," *Journal of Mental Science* 104 (1958): 1043-51; A. Binitie, "Psychiatric Disorders in a Rural Practice in the Bendel State of Nigeria," *Acta Psychiatrica Scandinavica* 64 (1981): 273-80; T. Harding, "Psychosis in a Rural West African Community," *Social Psychiatry* 8 (1973): 198-203; Timothy W. Harding, "Psychiatry in Rural Agrarian Societies," *Psychiatric Annals* 8 (1978): 302-10; David M. Ndetei and Joseph Muhangi, "The Prevalence and Clinical Presentation of Psychiatric Illness in a Rural Setting in Kenya," *British Journal of Psychiatry* 135 (1979): 269-72: David I. Ben-Tovim and Josephine M. Cushnie, "The Prevalence of Schizophrenia in a Remote Area of Botswana," *British Journal of Psychiatry* 148 (1986): 576-80.

Significant literature points to the psychopathology of African urban life: Peter C. W. Gutkind, "The Energy of Despair: Social Organization of the Unemployed in Two African Cities: Lagos and Nairobi," *Civilization* 17 (1967): 186-214, 380-405; A. Raymond Mills, "The Effects of Urbanization on Health in a Mining Area of Sierra Leone," *Transactions of the Royal Society of Tropical Medicine and Hygiene* 61 (1967): 114-30; Charles C. Hughes and John M. Hunter, "Disease and Development in Africa," *Social Science and Medicine* 3 (1970): 443-68. An important historical analysis on the social pathology of poverty is John Iliffe, *The African Poor: A History* (London: Cambridge University Press, 1987.

A large bibliography exists on drug and alcohol addiction in Africa: see O. I. Ifabumuyi, "Alcohol and Drug Addiction in Northern Nigeria," *Acta Psychiatrica Scandinavica* 73 (1986): 479-80; D. M. Ndetei, P. Kiptong, and K. Odhiambo, "Feighner's Symptom Profile of Alcoholism in a Kenyan General Hospital," *Acta Psychiatrica Scandinavica* 69 (1984): 409-15. For addiction and violent behavior, including suicide, see T. Asuni, "Suicide in Western Nigeria," *British Medical Journal* 3 (1962): 1091-96; H.N.K. arap Mengech and M. Dhadphale, "Attempted Suicide (Parasuicide) in Nairobi," *Acta Psychiatrica Scandinavica* 69 (1984): 416-19; Adego E. Eferakeya, "Drugs and Suicide Attempts in Benin City, Nigeria," *British Journal of Psychiatry* 145 (1984): 70-73; L. Jacobsson, "Acts of Violence in a Traditional Western Ethiopian Society in Transition," *Acta Psychiatrica Scandinavica* 72 (1985): 601-7.

Studies on traditional health care abound. A good survey of the changing views of the traditional healer is W. G. Jilek, "From Crazy Witch Doctor to Auxiliary Psychotherapist - The Changing Image of the Medicine Man," *Psychiatrica Clinica* 4 (1971): 200-20. An excellent work containing superb bibliographies is Z. A. Ademuwagun, J.A.A. Ayoade, I. E. Harrison, and D. M. Warren, eds., *African Therapeutic Systems* (Waltham, Mass.: Crossroads Press, 1979). Other important books are Leith Mullings, *Therapy, Ideology, and Social Change: Mental Healing in Urban Ghana* (Berkeley: University of California Press, 1984); John M. Janzen, *The Quest for Therapy in Lower Zaire* (Berkeley: University of California Press, 1978); Pascal James Imperato, *African Folk Medicine: Practices and Beliefs of the Bambara and Other Peoples* (Baltimore, Md.: York Press, 1977); Ari Kiev, ed., *Magic, Faith, and Healing: Studies in Primitive Psychiatry Today* (New York: Free Press, 1964); David Landy, ed., *Culture, Disease,and Healing: Studies in Medical Anthropology* (New York: Macmillan, 1977); Catherine M. Una Maclean, *Magical Medicine* (Edinburgh: University of Edinburgh Press, 1972); Anita Jacobson-Widding and David Westerlund, *Culture, Experience and Pluralism: Essays on African Ideas of Illness and Healing* (Uppsala: Almqvist & Wiksell International, 1989).

A growing body of literature stresses the importance of the traditional healer to a modern medical system: Gustav Jahoda, "Traditional Healers and Other Institutions Concerned with Mental Illness in Ghana," *International Journal of Social Psychiatry* 7 (1971): 245-68; Walter Otsyula, "Native and Western Healing: The Dilemma of East African Psychiatry," *Journal of Nervous and Mental Disease* 156 (1973): 297-99; Priscilla R. Ulin, "The Traditional Healer of Botswana in a Changing Society," *Rural Africana* 26 (1974): 123-30; Ira E. Harrison, "Traditional Healers: A Neglected Source of Manpower," *Rural Africana* 26 (1974): 5-16; A. O. Odejide, M. O. Olatawura, Okinade O. Sanda, and A. O. Oyeneye, "Traditional Healers and Mental Illness in the City of Ibadan," *Journal of Black Studies* 9 (1978): 195-205; Edward C. Green, "Roles for African Traditional Healers in Mental Health Care," *Medical Anthropology* 4 (1980): 489-522; Edward C. Green, "Can Collaborative Programs Between Biomedical and African Indigenous Health Practitioners Succeed?" *Social Science and Medicine* 27 (1988): 1125-30.

For good discussions on the political ramifications of Western medicine in non-Western areas of the world, see David Arnold, ed., *Imperial Medicine and Indigenous Societies* (Manchester: Manchester University Press, 1988); and Roy MacLeod and Milton Lewis, eds., *Disease, Medicine, and Empire: Perspectives on Western Medicine and the Experience of European Expansion* (London: Routledge, 1988).

Index

About the Author

LELAND V. BELL is Chair and Professor of History at Central State University in Wilberforce, Ohio. His most recent books are *Treating the Mentally Ill: From Colonial Times to the Present* (Praeger, 1980) and *Caring for the Retarded in America* (Greenwood Press, 1984).

Lightning Source UK Ltd.
Milton Keynes UK
UKOW06n0919070715

254704UK00013B/134/P